American Medical Asso(

Physicians dedicated to the health of Americ

The Handbook *of* Physician Health

The Essential Guide to Understanding the Health Care Needs of Physicians

Edited by

Larry S. Goldman, MD

Michael Myers, MD

Leah J. Dickstein, MD

The Handbook of Physician Health
The Essential Guide to
Understanding the Health Care Needs of Physicians

© 2000, American Medical Association
Printed in the United States of America.
All rights reserved.

Internet address: www.ama-assn.org

Additional copies of this book may be ordered from the American Medical Association. For order information, call toll-free 800 621-8335. Mention product number OP720399.

ISBN: 1-57947-004-1

BQ62:99-1369:1M:1/00

Table of Contents

Acknowledgments

We would like to thank everyone involved with this book for their hard work and efforts. Without their help, this book would not have been possible. In addition to those who wrote and contributed chapters, we would like to thank the people that volunteered their time and expertise to review the manuscript, specifically John Fromson, MD; Stanley G. Sataren, MD; G. Douglas Talbott, MD; Lynn Hankes, MD; Joan M. Brewster, PhD, and Daniel H. Angres, MD.

Chapter 1

Evolution of the Physician Health Field

Larry S. Goldman, MD,
Michael Myers, MD,
Leah J. Dickstein, MD

There have been ethical imperatives since antiquity urging physicians to steer clear of intemperate habits and to take care of themselves so that they were fit to look after patients. The modern beginnings of the physician health field, however, probably began in the 1960s with a number of studies showing that physicians were misusing alcohol and other drugs at a rate that suggested that these problems—and their attendant adverse effects on patient care—were more widespread than previously thought. Although there remained a continuing public and professional debate about whether those with addictions were truly ill or just morally defective, there was a growing consensus that it was better to try to treat (rehabilitate) physicians than to simply waste society's investment in them by drumming them out of the profession. So-called sick doctor statutes went on the books in Florida in 1969 and Texas in 1971 in an attempt to impose a regulatory structure for addressing this problem.

In 1972, the American Medical Association's (AMA's) Council on Mental Health published its report, "The Sick Physician," drawing the profession's and the public's attention to the problem of impaired physicians. The report noted the articles that had appeared in the medical literature during the preceding 15 to 20 years suggesting that substance abuse (including alcoholism), other mental disorders, and suicide were significant health problems among physicians. This AMA report called for (1) all physicians to take responsibility for impaired colleagues, (2) the referral of impaired colleagues to appropriate committees or boards in order to obtain treatment and to protect patients, (3) educational programs for medical trainees about these problems, and (4) the development and implementation of model legislation for states in dealing with impaired physicians.

This report catalyzed a period of increased legislative and regulatory activity, and it also led to the establishment of new programs to assess, treat, and/or monitor impaired physicians; new course offerings in medical schools and residencies to educate trainees and to attempt to "inoculate" them against these putative occupational hazards; and additional research to clarify the nature, risk factors, course, and outcomes for impaired physicians. During this time (1970s and early 1980s) most of this activity was focused on alcoholism and other substance abuse, and the emphasis was on physician impairment and recovery from these substance use disorders after they had already taken their toll. Eventually every state had developed some committee or program to deal with affected physicians, and as more physicians came forward (or were sent into these programs), more clinical and epidemiologic information began to accumulate.

First, subsequent studies of addiction rates among trainees and practicing physicians suggested that, overall, physicians' misuse of substances was not necessarily greater than that of nonphysicians of comparable age and other similar demographic factors. While rates of abuse of prescription drug use seemed to run somewhat higher, rates of illicit drugs were quite a bit lower. Second, there was a growing appreciation for the occurrence in physicians of other mental disorders, particularly depression and bipolar disorder. These conditions were seen both as co-occurrent with substance use disorders and as simply occurring by themselves. Finally, there were other conditions that caused impairment that were not mental disorders or at least that did not fit well into standard psychiatric nomenclature. In the first group were physical infirmities, including cardiac, musculoskeletal, neurologic (stroke, multiple sclerosis, blindness, etc), and other conditions. The second category consisted of behavioral problems such as sexual exploitation of patients or abusiveness toward patients or coworkers.

Many impaired physician programs were developed in conjunction with state medical societies. In some cases this was simply a small, voluntary committee of society members, but certain states began to develop more extensive programs with a professional staff and even medical directors. Some states have created "diversion programs," which allow physicians to be referred to health programs without having to be reported to their state licensing boards. States with those arrangements have generally found that they are able to get more physicians to enter treatment voluntarily, often at earlier stages of their illnesses (ie, before they were so impaired that they did something to warrant licensing board reporting or action).

As some of these programs came to enjoy the trust of their licensing boards and of individual physicians, the scope of types of cases coming to the programs widened. This expanded clinical demand—along with the research findings mentioned earlier—has led the field to a further shift from substance abuse and impairment alone to broader consideration of disorders of all types and incorporation of disease prevention and health promotion. The wellness movement* that has been growing in general medical practice has also been affecting the physician health movement as physicians have been urged to attend to areas of their life other than their medical careers.

In the past decade, as the health care delivery system has undergone profound changes, there has been more evidence than ever before of job dissatisfaction among physicians. This has been seen not only in survey data, but also by the greatly increased numbers of physicians going on medical disability, moving to nonclinical positions, taking early retirement, or leaving medicine entirely. These changes have led to new services being available for physicians in the areas of career renewal and counseling, retraining, and outplacement assistance. These various components of the physician health field are shown schematically in Figure 1-1 (page 4).

One question that people unfamiliar with the field of physician health often ask is why such a field exists. After all, the query goes,

---

* For example, increased appreciation of such things as social support networks, emotional health, spirituality, the doctor-patient relationship, and nontraditional healing methods on overall health and well-being.

Figure 1-1
Timeline of Aspects of Physician Health

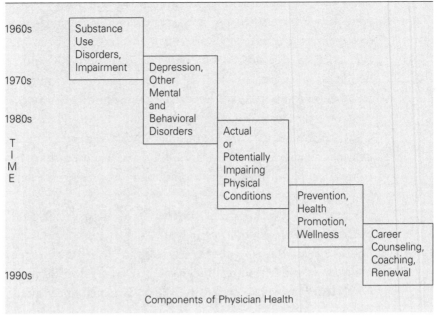

physicians enjoy far better income and access to care than the average citizen, so why expend resources studying and helping them? We feel that there are three reasons. First is the humanitarian one, namely that ameliorating suffering of everyone as much as possible is important. Second, there is a public health and patient safety reason: healthy physicians are far more likely to be helpful, effective doctors than those with unrecognized or untreated illnesses. And finally, society has made a tremendous investment in physician education and training: discarding rather than rehabilitating an ailing physician, when possible, is a squandering of this investment. Even physicians who do not have impairing conditions but are "only" stressed out, unhappy, distracted, or sleep deprived are more likely to make errors or unwise clinical decisions, and their patients may suffer.

As the field of physician health has continued to evolve, there has been an ongoing need to disseminate information about clinical practice, program development, and regulatory issues to practitioners, administrators, and educators. There are a number articles published every year, but these are widely scattered among many diverse journals,* making it difficult for someone to follow the field as a whole. One forum for the dissemination of new information has been a series of international conferences held every one to two years that are co-hosted by the AMA and the Canadian Medical Association. This book is intended as another such forum, designed to give the reader a broad exposure to the field of physician health and well-being.

The Handbook of Physician Health is intended as a broad introduction to the many facets of this field. It is intended for physicians and physicians-in-training, family members and loved ones of physicians and physicians-in-training, members of medical staff and medical society physician impairment committees, medical society alliance (auxiliary) members, hospital and managed care organization administrators and attorneys, members of licensing boards, and physicians caring for physician-patients. It is not intended as a scholarly tome based solely on research findings, nor is it confined to clinical material only. It is intended to be readable and practical, covering scientific, clinical, regulatory, and policy issues germane to many physician health-related topics. The emphasis is on helping readers to understand better the health care needs of physicians, the barriers to their getting appropriate care, and the ways to improve access and the care itself. The material draws on what is known about problem areas generally (eg, depression) but emphasizes what is unique to physicians alone or perhaps to physicians as part of a class (eg, high-status professionals, upper-bracket income earners, etc).

In Chapter 2 (Self-care, Prevention, and Health Promotion), Dr Frank (a preventive cardiologist) summarizes physicians' health and health behaviors, including their use of prevention strategies. In Chapter 3 (Physicians with Physical Disabilities), Drs Strax, Wainapel, and Welner (all physical medicine and rehabilitation specialists) review some of the most common physical conditions that can cause physicians difficulties in practicing, and they discuss some of the technical, environmental, and other strategies to minimize the impact of these conditions.

---

* Including general medical, substance abuse, psychiatry, academic medicine, physiatry, occupational medicine, state medical society, legal, and regulatory.

Chapters 4 through 9 examine what is known about the psychology of physicians and how this intersects with a number of well-documented psychiatric, emotional, and behavioral problems that some physicians exhibit. In Chapter 4 (Physician Temperament, Psychology, and Stress), Dr Notman (a psychiatrist) reviews the findings on personality traits that are especially common among physicians and the numerous stresses they face. She addresses the critical differences between male and female physicians and highlights special stresses for particular physician groups. In Chapter 5 (Physicians and Intimate Relationships), Dr Myers (a psychiatrist) looks at common problems physicians face in finding, establishing, and maintaining close relationships. He draws on his extensive practice of working clinically with partnerships, where one or both members are physicians, to show frequent pitfalls and offer solutions.

Dr Gautam (a psychiatrist) reviews anxiety and mood problems in physicians in Chapter 6 (Depression and Anxiety), highlighting the aspects of presentation and care that may differ when physicians are affected by these illnesses. Dr Silverman (a psychiatrist-suicidologist) reviews the demographics of physician suicide in Chapter 7, identifying established risk factors and offering both a preventive approach and clinical advice for caring for physicians where suicide is a higher-probability outcome. In Chapter 8, Drs Dilts and Gendel (both psychiatrist-addictionologists) summarize the broad literature of physician addictions, including risk factors, illness course, prognosis, and optimal approaches to assessment, monitoring, and treatment. Drawing on their own extensive experience at the Colorado Physician Health Program, they examine not only clinical care but how it is affected by regulatory issues. Dr Gendel reviews problematic physician behaviors in Chapter 9, particularly boundary transgressions and disruption (interpersonal difficulties with colleagues and other members of health care teams). He shows how important it is to evaluate the often-multiple causes of such problem behaviors, as the causes rather than the particular behaviors themselves generally influence treatment and prognosis.

In Chapter 10, Dr Dickstein (a psychiatrist) summarizes the special issues that are germane to medical students and residents, including stresses, clinical care, and administrative responses. She reviews curricular and program responses to prevent problems and/or assist troubled trainees. In Chapter 11, Dr Goldstein (a geropsychiatrist), looks at the other end of the developmental spectrum, examining the problems and rewards faced by aging physicians and how they are best understood and addressed. In Chapter 12, Dr Goldman (a consultation-liaison psychiatrist) summarizes how physicians react to becoming ill and how their "special" status as physicians can color their reaction—and the reactions of those around them—to an illness throughout its course.

Dr Van Komen (an internist with extensive licensing board experience) describes in Chapter 13 the various entities involved with oversight and review of physician impairment, the policy imperatives that provide their mandate, and how they carry out their administrative and regulatory duties. He emphasizes the interplay among different systems and the tensions that need to be resolved in many cases between appropriate protective and therapeutic approaches.

In Chapter 14, Dr Pearson (a pediatrician and career coach/counselor) goes over some of the forces that have created workplace dissatisfaction for physicians and the different ways that these dissatisfactions might be ameliorated by appropriate assessment and assistance. In Chapter 15, Drs Brown (a senior scientist with the AMA Physician Health Program) and Goldman have assembled a list of additional information sources and other resources for many aspects of physician health.

Each chapter of this book is intended to be a practical, readable reference on the topic covered that is based on the most current research and thinking. Any chapter can easily be read alone for those interested in that particular topic. There are suggested readings in each chapter for those readers who wish to explore a topic in greater depth.

Suggested General Readings

Brewster JM. Prevalence of alcohol and other drug problems among physicians. *JAMA*. 1986;255:1913.

Casper E, Dilts SL, Soter JJ, et al. Establishment of the Colorado physician health program with a legislative initiative. *JAMA*. 1988;260:671-673.

Corbet B, Madorsky JG. Physicians with disabilities. *West J Med*. 1991;154:514-521.

Council on Mental Health. The sick physician: impairment by psychiatric disorders, including alcoholism and drug dependence. *JAMA*. 1972;223:684-687.

Council on Scientific Affairs. *Substance Abuse Among Physicians*. Chicago: American Medical Association; 1995. Hughes PH, Brandenburg N, Baldwin DC. Prevalence of substance abuse among US physicians. *JAMA*. 1992;267:2333-2339.

Summer GL, McCrory E. Professional sexual misconduct. *Alabama Med*. 1994;64:4-6.

Ziegler PP. The physicians' health programs of the educational and scientific trust of the Pennsylvania Medical Society. *Fed Bull*. 1995;82:151-154.

Chapter 2

Self-care, Prevention, and Health Promotion

Erica Frank, MD, MPH

D o physicians practice what they preach and have relatively healthy personal habits, and can they expect, therefore, to live longer than do others? Does having healthful habits themselves make it more likely that physicians will discuss related preventive practices with their patients? Contrary to pervasive myths, the answer to all these questions is yes. This chapter will explore the facts and some of the myths about physician health.

Physicians' Personal General Health Practices

The Myths

When I began work on the Women Physicians' Health Study, many people said I'd find terrible health practices among women physicians. People said that because the study population was women, they would have so many duties, so many conflicts, and so much "role strain" that they would have poor self-care. This seemed like 19th-century thought, suggesting that if you overeducate a woman and give her too much professional responsibility, her reproductive organs would not function properly, but I had no hard data then to refute such thoughts. In addition to being women, many added, these individuals would have the heavy burden of being physicians, a group that some have called "ideal targets" for pathology and ill health. This also struck me as wrong and insulting to those nonphysicians who work long hours at unrewarding jobs for incomes that are only a fraction of physicians'; or those who derive neither job satisfaction nor a livelihood that permits their spouse to stay at home.

As explained below, these naysayers were wrong, but why would such myths have emerged? One major reason is that physicians, being human, do of course have some problems, and we take notice of and are understandably disturbed by the alcoholic physician, or the physician who smokes, or is morbidly obese: it suggests that, for whatever reasons, this physician doesn't practice what he or she should or does preach. Second, many of those who have written about physician health primarily interact with the small but disconcerting numerator of not-healthy physicians, and spend less time observing and reporting on the large healthy denominator. This is the classic "clinician's illusion" of mistakenly believing that those seen in general population samples are the same as those seen in their clinical samples.

Why does it matter if people incorrectly believe that physicians have poor health behaviors? We have shown that patients find that physicians with healthy personal practices are more credible and motivating. This is no surprise, for it is hard to imagine, for example, that a nonexercising physician could be an especially compelling advocate for exercise. It is time to put these false, toxic myths behind us.

The Facts

A fair amount is known about physicians' personal health practices, especially those of women physicians. The major data source for women physicians' practices is the Women Physicians' Health Study (WPHS), a representative, national study with 4,501 US respondents and 716 variables queried, conducted in 1993 to 1994. In general, women physicians reported healthy habits, exceeded national health goals for all examined behaviors, consistently had health-related behaviors better than those of the general population of women, and, in many cases, even outperformed other women of the highest socioeconomic status (SES).

Tobacco. Both men and women physicians' most obvious exemplary health behavior relates to cigarette smoking. Reported rates for both women and men physicians are now less than 4%, compared with about one quarter of those in the general population. As shown in Table 2-1, compared with women in the general population, women physicians were one seventh as likely to smoke, half as likely ever to have been smokers, and, if they had smoked, were nearly twice as likely to have quit.

Table 2-1
Health Practices of Women Physicians in the United States

Characteristic	Not High SES[a]	High SES[a]	Physicians
Cigarette smoking			
Smoking history			
Never	52.9 (0.4)*	64.0 (1.9)*	77.7 (0.7)
Former smoker	22.1 (0.3)*	28.0 (1.8)*	18.6 (0.7)
Current	25.0 (0.4)*	8.0 (1.0)*	3.7 (0.4)
Mean age at onset, yr[b]	18.8 (0.1)*	18.9 (0.3)	19.6 (0.7)
Mean no. of cigarettes/day[b]	17.6 (0.2)*	16.0 (0.2)	12.0 (1.1)
≥ 1 cigarette-abstinent days in last yr, %[b]	50.5 (0.9)*	47.0 (6.1)*	75.3 (4.0)
No. of years quit, %[c]			
<1	11.9 (0.5)*	6.7 (2.1)	3.5 (0.8)
1-4	20.8 (0.7)*	14.0 (2.3)	16.2 (1.7)
≥ 5	67.3 (0.8)*	79.3 (2.9)	80.3 (1.9)
Alcohol consumption			
Drinking in past month, %	43.9 (0.4)*	63.3 (1.9)*	72.4 (0.9)
Mean drinking, days/mo[d]	6.1 (0.1)*	7.2 (0.3)**	8.5 (0.2)
Mean no. of drinks/episode[d]	2.0 (0.0)*	1.6 (0.0)*	1.4 (0.0)
Mean no. of episodes/mo of >4 drinks[d]	0.4 (0.0)*	0.1 (0.0)	0.1 (0.0)
Other			
Mean fruit and vegetable score	3.3 (0.0)*	3.8 (0.1)**	3.5 (0.0)
Mean block dietary fat score	27.3 (0.3)*	21.6 (0.9)	24.1 (0.3)
Seatbelt wearing, %			
Always or nearly always	85.5 (0.3)*	95.1 (0.8)	96.3 (0.4)
Sometimes or seldom	11.3 (0.3)*	4.5 (0.8)	3.3 (0.4)
Never	3.2 (0.2)*	0.4 (0.2)	0.4 (0.1)

Note: All figures shown are age-standardized point estimates (± standard error) in women. Adapted from Frank E, Brogan DJ, Mokdad AH, et al. Health-related behaviors of women physicians vs other women in the United States. *Arch Intern Med.* 1998;158:342-348.

[a] Data from Behavioral Risk Factor Surveillance System (BRFSS); SES, socioeconomic status.
[b] Current smokers only.
[c] Former smokers only.
[d] Only includes those who consumed alcohol in past month.

*P<0.001 for the difference between BRFSS item and women physicians.
**P<0.01 for the difference between BRFSS item and women physicians.

Alcohol. Both data from WPHS and other data show that physicians are less likely to abstain from alcohol than are other women and men in the general population. However, although only one quarter of women and men physicians reported complete abstinence in the past month, women physicians who consumed alcohol reported drinking on average only twice a week, consuming less per episode of drinking than did other women drinkers, and reporting almost never drinking large amounts. The differential between physician and lay alcohol abstinence rates may reflect physicians' assessments of current scientific opinion on alcohol consumption (as well as their personal recreational preferences), since the contemporary medical literature generally supports the safety of low alcohol consumption along with the harmfulness of high consumption.

Diet. Men physicians' dietary habits have not been well examined, but women physicians eat somewhat more fruits and vegetables and less fat than did less-advantaged women, and somewhat fewer fruits and vegetables and more fat than other high-SES women (see Table 1). One third define themselves as overweight: nearly all of these physicians report trying to lose weight, and they do so by trying to change their exercise and eating habits. Personal histories of eating disorders and obesity are uncommon (<10%). Most women physicians never drink whole milk, two thirds never eat hot dogs, and about half never eat cold cuts or butter.

Exercise. Men physicians' exercise habits have also not been well examined, but nearly all women physicians (96%) reported some exercise performance, and the median amount of time spent exercising was 3 hours per week. The most common form of exercise was walking, followed by gardening, biking, "other," swimming, running, and aerobics. Although nearly all women physicians report performing some exercise, only half comply with the recommendation to exercise 30 minutes or more, at least 3 times per week. Women physicians 60 years and older, those with female personal physicians, and unmarried women physicians complied with the exercise recommendations at somewhat higher rates, and nonwhites had significantly lower compliance rates than whites. Number of hours worked was not associated with compliance rates.

Health screening. Though not extensively tested, physicians' health screening practices also seem to be better than those of the general population. Nearly 90% have had their cholesterol tested in the past five years, and, of those older than 50 years, three fourths have had fecal occult blood testing and about half have had sigmoidoscopy. They may not, however, have more screening than other individuals of high SES; this has not been well studied in men physicians.

Physician Mortality

What do these healthy behaviors translate into in terms of rates of disease and death among physicians? We have found (manuscript in review) that for both white and black men, physicians are older at death when compared with others in the population, with all examined professionals, and specifically with lawyers. Since the number of physicians has increased dramatically in recent years (nearly doubling, for example, between 1970 and 1990), this is especially impressive, as such a trend makes available a relatively high proportion of young physicians who could die, increases the statistical contribution of younger physicians dying, and lowers the average age at death. Because the increase in numbers of women physicians has been particularly large, though (with the number of women medical school graduates increasing nearly ninefold between 1950 and 1990), analyses of women physicians' average age at death is not meaningful.

It is noteworthy that, while black male physicians die later than do other blacks, they nonetheless die younger than do white male non-professionals. While it may be a function of blacks' higher general mortality rates, it may also be at least partly due to the relatively recent increase in admissions of black males to non–historically black medical schools, again increasing the statistical impact of younger black physicians dying.

It is not surprising that physicians die at older ages than do others, given the healthy worker effect (ie, that those who can work may be healthier than those who do not or cannot), physicians' high SES, and the data shown previously demonstrating that physicians tend to make healthy choices. However, since one can compare physician data with that of other professionals, it is possible to decrease the confounding nature of the healthy worker effect and of physicians' higher SES. What remains are two possibilities: that healthier individuals choose medicine, and/or that individuals who have received medical training make healthier choices (as we have seen above) and therefore have lower mortality rates.

Other studies that have directly examined US physician mortality have also found lower cumulative rates. Williams and colleagues compared mortality data from the Harvard Medical School graduating classes between 1923-1924, 1932-1934, and 1942-1944 with data from other age-matched US white men, and found lower cumulative mortality for the physicians. A study of physician graduates of the University of Southern California and Loma Linda University found that both groups had standardized mortality ratios lower than that of age-matched white men (and the predominantly Adventist/vegetarian Loma Linda graduates had standardized mortality rates [SMRs] even lower than that of the University of Southern California graduates, 56 versus 76). A 1969 to 1973 study of physician mortality reported to the AMA Masterfile found SMRs of 75 for men and 84 for women physicians; a 1980 to 1988 study of young US physicians whose deaths were reported in *JAMA* found SMRs less than half that of the same-age general population. Such findings are also echoed by a 1971 to 1980 Finnish study in which physicians had lower comparative mortality figures than did other workers and by those of a large, comprehensive British survey examining deaths between 1962 and 1992, in which the SMR of the physicians was less than half that expected (SMR, 48; 95% confidence interval, 46-49).

Why Does Physician Health Matter?

While it may be good for physicians that they have healthy habits, should this matter to anyone else? In fact, physicians' personal health habits may strongly affect their clinical practices, a matter of concern to every patient or potential patient.

In the Women Physicians' Health Study, personal related health habits were shown to affect physicians' likelihood to report counseling or screening patients regarding cholesterol, exercise, alcohol use, smoking cessation, flu vaccine, breast and skin cancer prevention and detection, and use of hormonal replacement therapy. Prior mixed-gender analyses of physician behavior have also shown that physicians who themselves have healthy personal habits are more likely to encourage their patients to adopt such habits. Specifically, these smaller trials have shown that regular exercisers are more likely to counsel their patients on exercise habits; nonsmokers to counsel on smoking; seatbelt users to counsel on seatbelt use; and low-fat food eaters and those who themselves have been screened for cholesterol to counsel on cholesterol.

Why might a physician with healthy personal practices be more likely to counsel or screen patients about related practices? Such physicians could be more interested in prevention and may therefore extend their personal interests into the clinical context. They might be better able to address barriers to, benefits from, and costs of behavior change, or be more knowledgeable about the physiologic effects of behavior change. For example, those who adhere to a low-fat diet could suggest ways in which they have overcome social pressures to eat poorly, highlight their pleasure with the concomitant weight loss that often accompanies lower-fat diets, recommend inexpensive local restaurants that serve healthy options, and discuss their increased stamina when hiking local trails. Physicians with high personal investment in healthy habits thus not only are more active preventionists, but, as discussed above, are also more effective. Personal health practices may also interact with perceived counseling relevance, self-confidence in performing counseling/screening, and even amount of training in a topic, three areas that are highly related to counseling frequency.

Suggested Readings

Bortz WM. Health behavior and experiences of physicians: results of a survey of Palo Alto Medical Clinic physicians. *West J Med*. 1992;156:50-51.

Frank E. The Women Physicians' Health Study: background, objectives, and methods. *J Am Med Womens Assoc*. 1995;50:64-66.

Frank E, Brogan DJ, Mokdad AH, Simoes EJ, et al. Health-related behaviors of women physicians vs other women in the United States. *Arch Intern Med*. 1998;158:342-348.

Glanz K, Fiel SB, Walker LR, Levy MR. Preventive health behavior of physicians. *J Med Educ*. 1982;57:637-639.

Hensrud DD, Sprafka JM. The smoking habits of Minnesota physicians. *Am J Public Health*. 1993;83:415-417.

Hughes PH, Brandenburg N, Baldwin DC Jr, Storr CL, WilHams KM, Sheehan DV. Prevalence of substance use among US physicians [published correction appears in *JAMA*. 1992;268:2518]. JAMA. 1992;267:2333-2339.

Nelson DE, Glovino GA, Emont SL, et al. Trends in cigarette smoking among US physicians and nurses. *JAMA*. 1994;271:1273-1275.

Schwartz JS, Lewis CE, Clancy C, Kinosian MS, Radany MH, Koplan JP. Internists' practices in health promotion and disease prevention: a survey. *Ann Intern Med*. 1991;114:46-53.

Wells KB, Lewis CE, Leake B, Ware JE Jr. Do physicians preach what they practice? A study of physicians' health habits and counseling practices. *JAMA*. 1984;252:2846-2848.

Williams SV, Munford RS, Colton T, Murphy DA, Poskanzer DC. Mortality among physicians: a cohort study. *J Chronic Dis*. 1971;24:393-401.

Wyshak G, Lamb GA, Lawrence RS, Curran WJ. A profile of the health-promoting behaviors of physicians and lawyers. *N Engl J Med*. 1980;303:104-107.

Chapter 3

Physicians with Physical Disabilities

Thomas E. Strax, MD,
Stanley F. Wainapel, MD, MPH,
Sandra Welner, MD

T o be born with a disability or to acquire a disability in life places you in a very special group. Suddenly, you become less worthy, less important, less deserving. *Disability* means that you do not have ability. Throughout childhood we were brought up to believe that people with disabilities were less intelligent and emotionally and morally deprived. These people were not deserving of our attention, our praise, or our money. Even professional people with a disability were suspect. A physician who developed Parkinson's disease might be assumed to be an alcoholic with the shakes. An individual suffering from a stroke, multiple sclerosis, visual loss, hearing loss, or even heart disease may be viewed as someone who could no longer be trusted to perform adequately in his or her chosen field. Tringo[1] in 1970 investigated the attitudes of non disabled high school students, college undergraduates, college graduate students, and rehabilitation workers to some 21 specific disabilities. He found that the subjects with higher education levels showed less rejection of individuals with disabilities. There were nine possible ratings from which to choose that range varied from "would marry" to "would put to death." The highest-ranking brain-injured type was epilepsy, and that ranked only 13th out of 21.[2]

This chapter will explore some of these issues and attitudes and ways that, with small accommodations, people with disabilities can do whatever they need to do in the health care profession. The chapter will first examine what is known about the epidemiology of disabilities and then look at particular assistive strategies. It will then review the particular problems and solutions at each stage of the physician's career pathway.

Epidemiology of Physical Disabilities Among Physicians

Approximately 17% of noninstitutionalized Americans have a physical disability when this is defined as *any limitation of usual or appropriate life activities due to a chronic health condition or impairment*.[3] The comparable prevalence rate of physical disabilities among American physicians is not known, since similar detailed surveys have not been made in this population. Lewis[4] has suggested a prevalence of 4% and Martini[5] quoted a prevalence of 2.5%, but both figures are only estimates without supporting surveillance data. An unpublished survey by the American Medical Association of 1,000 physicians randomly selected from the Los Angeles County Medical Association found that 52 (10.1%) of the 510 respondents reported having at least one physical disability.

An analysis of 259 physicians and medical students compiled from inquiries received by the American Society of Handicapped Physicians during a three-year period and reported by Wainapel[6] represent the largest currently published study of the characteristics of physicians with physical disabilities. However, these data reflect considerable selection bias in favor of those with more severe and "visible" conditions and individuals more inclined to be members of a support organization.

This survey consisted of 211 men and 48 women with a median age of 42.5 years. It included 33 medical students and 26 resident physicians. Of the physicians surveyed, 75.3% were in active practice. The eight most frequently encountered disabilities were traumatic paraplegia/quadriplegia (41), multiple sclerosis (22), stroke syndromes (two), postpolio weakness (18), lower-extremity amputation (nine), diabetic retinopathy (nine), retinitis pigmentosa (eight), and systemic lupus erythematosus/connective tissue disease (eight). These diagnoses accounted for two thirds of the entire sample. Spinal cord injury was also the most common diagnosis in the medical student group (15 of 33). The five most frequent medical specialties were internal medicine (39), family practice (32), psychiatry (26), rehabilitation medicine (17), and pediatrics (17). Three disabilities-specialty "clusters" were identified: (1) visual impairment and psychiatry, (2) traumatic quadriplegia and radiology, and (3) diabetic retinopathy and internal medicine/family practice.

The data from this survey are of considerable interest. They show that a wide range of physical disabilities is represented among physicians and that continued medical practice is possible in spite of their occurrence. The higher than expected representation of rehabilitation medicine among specialities reflects the fact that physiatry has individuals with disabilities as its patient base and would therefore be particularly sensitive to the capacities or needs of practitioners with such disabilities. The predominance of cognitive rather than physical demand in psychiatric practice also makes psychiatry a more accessible specialty for physicians with visual impairment or blindness. The unexpected clustering of quadriplegia and radiology becomes more plausible when one considers that radiology departments are wheelchair accessible and have extensive support personnel who can function as physician extenders; moreover, the increasing availability of voice-activated computer software would simplify the process of dictating radiology reports for physicians with limited use of the hands.

The contrast between the data in Wainapel's study and the data in the unpublished AMA-sponsored Los Angeles County Medical Association survey is particularly striking. The latter group had a median age of 65 years, and the most frequent diagnoses were cardiovascular and pulmonary diseases. Thus, we are presented with a kind of epidemiologic iceberg in which the smaller portion of physicians with disabilities is more evident by virtue of the highly visible nature of their disorders (it is difficult to conceal the presence of paralysis, blindness, or joint deformities), while the far larger portion goes unrecognized because their disabilities (such as hearing loss or heart disease) are less visible and therefore easier to conceal. The hidden portion of this iceberg is particularly important in the older physician, who may develop one or more of the disabilities associated with the aging process.

Attitudes and Other Sociologic Issues

The distinction between "visible" and "invisible" disability has major implications not only for epidemiologic studies but also for its sociologic consequences. Physicians with less obvious disabilities will be understandably concerned about the stigma associated with such disabilities and will therefore conceal them by trying to "pass" as totally able-bodied. Their concern is justifiable based on the negative attitudes toward individuals with disabilities displayed by society as a whole and by physicians themselves. Lewis[4] cogently outlined these attitudes and the dilemmas they pose for a doctor with less obvious disability:

1. Society views individuals with disabilities as inferior and unproductive.

2. Physicians as members of society tend to show this attitude, but they also view disability as a failure of medical care since it is often not curable. This leads to the physician's attitude that "permanent," "incurable," and "terminal" are synonymous.

3. Society accords physicians a high level of status.

4. Physicians reflect this attitude by viewing themselves as having a high social status.

The physician who has a physical disability is thus simultaneously a member of a group perceived negatively by society and the medical community (disabled people) and a member of a positively perceived group (physicians). The conflicting status levels interfere with the acceptance by nondisabled physicians of their colleagues with disabilities. Such attitudinal barriers are often more difficult to overcome than the more tangible ones posed by nonaccessible architecture or environments.[7]

With the passage of the Americans with Disabilities Act (ADA) in 1990, greater acceptance of physical differences has emerged. Frequently, this legal validation has not been translated into psychosocial equality. It is difficult to legislate attitudes and prejudicial assumptions held by many segments of society about how a competent, qualified individual should appear, walk, move, see, hear, etc. Physicians may be even more reluctant to accept these differences in colleagues because disability and physical difference are equated with the patient's role rather than that of the provider.[8, 9]

Men and women choose medical careers for a variety of reasons, most altruistic of which is the desire to help others by improving their health through the specialized knowledge of medicine. The decision to dedicate a lifetime to cure and comfort the ill may begin with a personal experience such as an illness in the family or the recognition of a special talent, ability, or interest. With this, the student begins to assume the identity of the healer.

However, when the healer is ill or disabled, it may be difficult for society and medical colleagues to reconcile these disparate images,[10] and how can a disabled physician grapple with irony in which he or she needs to be healed? How can physicians, traditionally viewed as healthy and physically able, maintain their self-image even when they can no longer walk, use their hands, hear, or see? Do these impairments render them less qualified as healers?

The television portrayal of the omnipotent doctor running to the aid of patients in distress is an image we have all grown up with and maintained, including those entering the field of medicine. Very few patients have been treated by physicians with disabilities, but usually the first startled look turns, in time, to trust with a demonstration of that doctor's competence and the patient's recognition of a disabled person's unique capacity to empathize. However, these physicians' own colleagues may associate the disability with a lack of qualification or an incapacity to perform skillfully, and therefore may not regard these professionals as worthy of practicing medicine or competing with other physicians for patients.[11] Before 1990, impairment in physicians was typically linked to substance abuse or mental illness. Clearly, if these disorders go untreated, a physician's judgment and competence can be affected. However, labeling physicians with such difficulties as "impaired" established an umbrella under which all physicians with a variety of impairments were grouped together.[12] Thus, physicians whose physical disabilities did not affect cognitive function or judgment were not differentiated in terminology from others with conditions that were more likely to impact on performance quality.[13]

Succeeding in all subspecialties, however, requires the ability to absorb enormous quantities of data, grasp the pertinent medical information, and apply it appropriately. A physical disability does not alter this capacity. Disability may, however, affect the practice of certain types of medicine. For example, a pathologist who loses vision will have a difficult time continuing to practice but may still contribute through education and research. Specialists who have a physical disability and are in the primary care specialty of internal medicine, pediatrics, or gynecology may continue their work by delegating specific physical tasks to others. Thus, these physicians may not need to lose their identities as healers, but simply modify their activities so they can still accomplish the goal of improving the health and knowledge of their patients and continue to contribute to the field.

Rehabilitation Strategies: Assistive Technology and Personal Assistance

Physicians with physical disabilities can draw upon a wealth of technologic and personal resources to maintain, establish, or reestablish their professional careers. The rapid advancements in adaptive technology that have revolutionized the lives of individuals with disabilities can similarly have a profound impact for these physicians. Such devices can range from the most simple and inexpensive to the highly complex and costly. Some specific examples will help to illustrate the crucial role that they can play.

Neuromuscular Disabilities

Neuromuscular disabilities such as spinal cord injury, multiple sclerosis, stroke, cerebral palsy, postpolio weakness, or severe arthritis may force a physician or medical student to use a wheelchair for all or most activities. The first requirement for such a physician is a wheelchair-accessible environment; this entails having building entrances with ramps, doors that can be easily opened or open automatically, and rooms with doors wide enough to fit the wheelchair. If all these factors are in place, one must still deal with issues such as examination tables lacking controls to adjust their height. This can severely hamper the physician's ability to do a physical examination from his/her wheelchair. Some simple devices such as a long-handled reflex hammer or stethoscope with elongated tubing can ease the examination under these circumstances. A special wheelchair that allows the user to stand up can also give the physician a better opportunity to perform maneuvers such as abdominal palpation and pelvic exam or even to help at surgical procedures. For those with back problems, there are special chairs for the operating room. Assistive technology centers exist across the country, each specializing in different kinds of adaptive equipment. The interested reader can contact these centers directly.

When hand function is compromised by weakness, ataxia, or joint deformity, the use of voice-activated computer software can enable the physician to dictate notes and reports even if unable to hold or operate a conventional Dictaphone. Similar software has been used in radiology departments for all physicians regardless of their physical status. Physician extenders such as nurse practitioners, physician assistants, or technicians (eg, in radiology) are invaluable assets, particularly when the physician has upper- and lower-extremity involvement. New robotics can also be used to aid physicians with diminished hand function. Even simple things like a Kelley clamp can be used instead of forceps to help hold a skin flap.

Visual Impairment

Visual impairment or blindness may not affect a physician's functions such as palpation, percussion, or auscultation, and a history can be elicited from the patient and recorded without undue difficulty by means of a good memory or a simple cassette recorder. However, observation, review of written materials or x-rays, writing, and performance of many vision-dependent activities become problematic. Adaptive technology for vision enhancement or substitution[14] can often eliminate or at least reduce these issues. Low-vision aids include magnifiers held in the hand, placed over objects, or hung around the user's neck. The less portable and more expensive closed-circuit television video magnifier (CCTV) can enlarge images from three to 60 times normal size and can also enhance color contrast through a reverse image on a black background. The CCTV is particularly helpful for individuals with low vision who need assistance with reading. When vision is too impaired for even the CCTV, it is possible to read printed material by using sophisticated optical-character recognition and synthetic speech software along with a computer and scanner. Screen-reading software is also available to enable blind physicians to have access to most material by computer, including medical literature and the Internet.

"Talking" technology, used for the talking thermometer, glucometer, and sphygmomanometer, is frequently a valuable aid. Medical textbooks are also available in recorded cassette format from Recordings for the Blind and Dyslexic of Princeton, New Jersey. Visually impaired physicians can also privately hire readers for use in their office or can use other personnel such as secretaries for this purpose.

Hearing Impairment

Specially adapted devices for physicians who have significant hearing impairment or deafness are invaluable aids to clinical practice. Likewise, closed-captioning of videotaped educational materials renders them accessible to such physicians. Interpreters may be required in hospital or office settings, but the combined use of hearing aids and a high degree of skill in lip-reading may suffice for many individuals.

Special Issues Along the Career Development Path

Medical School

What do we do with the individual with a disability who wishes to become a physician? It is one thing to make some accommodation for the colleague with an acquired disability, but should we admit someone who is less than "perfect" into medical school? There should be rules! We are a nation that prides itself on a national principle of equal opportunity and fair play for all. Unfortunately, in practice, the *all* means people who look like us and talk like us. Anybody who varies from our norm is less worthy and therefore less worthy of being given an equal opportunity. These people include those with impairments, health problems, and physical, mental and emotional disabilities.

It has taken many, many years for our country and its educational institutions to realize the merits and responsibilities of providing role models for minorities. These role models have given minorities the chance to say "why not?" and take up the challenge to improve themselves. The *New York Times* on September 18, 1995, published an editorial in which General Colin Powell pointed out that many of his Republican friends felt that it was time to eliminate "affirmative action," which was begun because of vague and ancient wrongs. General Powell said there is nothing vague about discrimination. Many minorities educated by the army return with a sense of pride to their communities and become role models for undereducated and unmotivated youth. People with disabilities are the second largest minority group, second only to women. There is a wonderful opportunity to use these individuals as useful members in our society, even in the healing arts.

Admission to medical school, however, to someone with a disability is a complicated and at times disappointing story. One reason for this discrimination has to do with semantics. Many people wrongly equate having a disability with being *handicapped.* The word handicapped comes from England and stands for "cap in hand," to signify the physically disabled beggar who cannot do anything and needs alms from good-natured individuals. Reasonable accommodations for students as for practicing physicians are important. Quite often individuals with so called "technical deficits" receive automatic rejection instead of exploration of appropriate accommodations.

On applying for admission to medical school, one of us (Dr Strax) was asked by the interviewer, "How dare you apply, don't you know there are people without disabilities trying to get into medical school?" Back in 1963, there were no guidelines on physical disabilities. Dr Strax was an experience and an experiment. The only other person with cerebral palsy who attended medical school, Dr Earl Carlson, did so in the 1920s. He was required to sign a contract saying that he would never ever see patients, only do research. We do not know if this was a true story, but we have been told that Dr Carlson tore up the contract. He went on to be one of the founders of the Neurological Institute at Columbia Presbyterian Medical School.

Between 1963, when Dr Strax entered medical school, and 1971, when he completed his residency, he was able to accomplish almost everything required with some minor adaptations, patience, help from classmates, and small accommodations by the school. During that time he delivered 14 babies. He also performed several lumbar punctures, helped in surgery, worked on the wards, and even did a closed liver biopsy. Most people were very helpful. However, there was an ex-Green Beret resident who felt that it was his job to weed out individuals whom *he* felt should not be physicians. The dean himself, who strongly opposed Dr Strax's admission, four years later stopped him in the hall to tell him that he had been wrong. Dr Strax was fortunate to have been given a chance. He owed this chance to Dr Howard Rusk, who fought with the faculty at New York University School of Medicine to give Strax, an individual with cerebral palsy, an opportunity to prove that he could, or could not, succeed in medical school.

Years later, as a faculty member at Temple University, Dr Strax supervised a medical student named David Hartman, who was blind. Dr Strax sent him and another medical student to see a patient who had severe scleroderma. Both medical students independently completed a history and examined the patient. Hartman identified that the patient had calcium extruding from her fingertips, a finding missed by the student with eyesight. Hartman also saw a patient on the trauma service with multiple fractures and injuries to both lower extremities. He identified that the patient also had bilateral ulnar nerve injuries; this was missed by the sighted attending physician and by the orthopedic residents.[*]

Robert Babcock, MD (1851-1930), who blinded himself while playing with a toy at age 13, became one of America's first distinguished physicians who had a disability. He compensated for his visual problems with incredible memory and with the use of other visual and nonvisual resources that were available to him. Like David Hartman, he mastered the ability to identify structures in a cadaver by feel.

A survey of 117 American medical schools in 1982 found that 39 schools had admitted at least one student with a disability during the 4-year period of the study. Of the 72 students, 40 did well or very well academically; 64 did well or very well interpersonally. Schools that had accepted one student with a disability tended to accept more of them. The most common diagnosis was spinal cord injury requiring the use of a wheelchair. Limb amputations, visual problems, and hearing loss led the list. Wainapel[6] included 33 disabled students in his study of 259 physicians with disabilities. Almost half of these students had spinal cord injuries as the cause of their physical disability. The second most common was hearing loss, which constituted five of the 33 disabilities.

Medical schools face the decision of whether to admit applicants with disabilities. This decision is left to a small committee of individuals with academic and clinical backgrounds. Few have real experience and understand what these students could accomplish

---

[*]Goethe once said:
   "We see what we are looking for
   We look for what we know
   What we don't know
   We never see."

with minor alterations to the environment and minimum accommodations. With advances in modern medicine, there will be an increase in the number of individuals with disabilities who survive their injuries and illnesses, apply to medical school, and become physicians.

American medical schools have been wrestling for many years with defining standards needed to be a medical student. In 1979, a special advisory panel of the Association of American Medical Colleges set up technical standards recommending motor, conceptual, integrative, quantitative, behavioral, and social guidelines for admission to American medical schools. This report was not a policy statement but was intended to be used as a guide for medical schools, which were supposed to establish their own technical standards. Ironically, over the years the principles have been used to *prevent* talented individuals with disabilities from attending American medical schools.

All medical schools are obligated to produce effective, competent, and compassionate physicians who will be best able to serve the needs of society. All professional schools should educate a diverse group of students, recognizing that in diversity lies excellence. Included in this diverse group are qualified students who have disabilities. Applicants with disabilities should, of course, be held to the same admission standards (with appropriate accommodations if needed for them to meet the admission standards) as their nondisabled peers.

Graduating medical students do not all enter the same field and therefore are not all pluripotential. Each field requires a different psychological, emotional, verbal, intellectual, and technical skill set. There are, of course, certain basic technical skills that may be essential and therefore must be gained by all medical students with or without the assistance of reasonable accommodations. There are some fields that not all physicians can enter because they require certain technical skills that many able-bodied medical students do not have. Therefore, candidates, even the able-bodied candidates, with compromised skills may not be suited for some of these specialties and should therefore be counseled by the school not to enter these fields. Each medical school should develop a written policy that guides the selection of students with disabilities. This policy should be regularly reviewed in light of continued changes in technology. Let us explore some of these requirements.

Observation. All medical students can get required information presented through demonstrations and experiences in basic sciences. This information is conveyed through physiologic and pharmacologic demonstrations in animals, microbiologic cultures, and microscopic images in normal and pathologic tissues. Much of this information is given in laboratories and lecture series, and a candidate would have to be able to glean this information in some way. Furthermore, candidates have to be able to observe a patient accurately at a distance and nearby. Candidates must find information from written documents and visual information presented in images from paper, slide, and video. Such observation and information acquisition usually require the functional use of visual, auditory and somatic sensation. In cases where a candidate's ability to observe or find information through sensory modalities is compromised, the candidates must show alternate means and/or abilities to find and show the essential information conveyed in this fashion. Medical schools should help students where necessary.

Communication. It is important that medical students show the ability to communicate verbal and written material effectively, efficiently, and sensitively with patients, their families, and all members of their health care team. This can be through traditional or alternative means. Medical students and physicians must also be able to accurately elicit information and describe a patient's change in mood, thought, activity, and posture. There are many accommodations and technical equipment that could be offered to a student to allow him/her to have effective communication skills.

Motor skills. Medical students and physicians should possess the motor skills necessary to do palpation, percussion, auscultation, and other diagnostic maneuvers and to perform basic laboratory tests and diagnostic procedures. It is also desirable for candidates to be able to execute motor movements required to provide general and emergency medical care, such as airway management, placement of intravenous catheters, cardiopulmonary resuscitation, and suturing of wounds. However, the candidate who cannot perform these tasks independently should at least be able to understand and direct another individual in the methodology involved in doing these activities. There are many established physicians in practice who have forgotten how to do emergency surgery or other skills that they had acquired in medical school. Shouldn't we prefer a physician who could direct another individual how to competently perform a life-saving procedure to one who did not know what he or she was doing?

Intellectual-conceptual, integrative, and qualitative abilities. Problem solving is a critical skill demanded of all physicians. It requires the use of all his or her intellectual abilities. Either directly, or with some accommodations, all students must be able to measure, calculate, reason, analyze, and synthesize. In addition, they should understand spatial and three-dimensional relationships. These must be comprehended with or without appropriate accommodations in a timely fashion. Intelligent, mature students with the ability to understand and integrate material should not be prevented from attending a medical school simply because they have a disability.

Behavioral and social attributes. Medical students and physicians must possess the emotional health required to exercise good judgment and promptly complete all responsibilities needed for diagnosis and care of patients. They should be able to develop mature, sensitive, and effective relationships with patients, families, and other health care providers. Students must be able to tolerate physically taxing workloads and function effectively under stress. Adaptation to changing environments is critical. One must display flexibility and be able to function in the face of the uncertainties inherent in the clinical care of patients. Compassion, integrity, concern for others, interpersonal skills, interest, and motivation are all personal qualities that should be assessed during the admission and educational process.

To meet these challenges and allow capable individuals with disabilities to train as physicians, each medical school must review its facility's environment to afford reasonable accommodations. All students must be able to access learning settings such as laboratories and clinical environments. Minor modifications and adaptations, such as ramps for access to buildings and viewing clinical activities, or laboratory procedures, are appropriate. Electric doors, handrails in hallways, and modifications of bathrooms are appropriate and required under the law. Furniture and furnishings should be appropriate for students who have disabilities. Occasionally, modifications in chairs, transcribing equipment, or special equipment for individuals with visual or hearing impairments should be available. There must be reasonable access to allow building-to-building transit, entrance, egress, and in-building mobility. Bathrooms and other public facilities, such as drinking fountains, telephones, and work surfaces, may need modifications. Some students who live on campus may also need housing accommodations.

One major resistance has been to the cost of appropriate accommodations. The costs of these reasonable accommodations should be shared by both the school and the student. A second problem concerns bias of faculty and other students. All schools should develop programs to sensitize and familiarize faculty, staff, and other students to reduce the level of misunderstanding or negative bias.

All schools should have a policy in place that deals with individuals with disabilities who might apply for admission. Applicants who believe they have not received adequate consideration because of their impairment or disability should be afforded the opportunity to appeal to a committee of the medical school that would review the appeal on a case-by-case basis. The ADA extends civil rights to people with disabilities. A paradigm shift is called for; a change in how we view things is necessary. Our ability to recognize these biases and understand our paradigms enables us to rationally address new situations. Failure to do this can limit our capacity to distinguish *ability* from *disability*. In considering our paradigm shift, it is vital to understand that the *function* of the individual with a disability, physician or otherwise, is far more important than the *diagnosis* of that individual.

Residency Training

The impact of a disability on a physician depends on the type of disability and the stage of the physician's career when it develops. If the condition is evident during the process of choosing a career path, the student can preselect a specialty that would be least likely to challenge any particular limitation and highlight the strengths. Previously, physicians with disabilities were discouraged from entering residency, as their limitations were viewed as incompatible with call schedules and the long hours required for adequate training. These perceptions by residency program coordinators may have been easily changed through creative problem solving incorporating suggestions from the physician-in-training.

Unfortunately, in the past, solutions like these were not carried out, and residency training was rarely made available to young physicians with disabilities. For example, Lisa Iezzoni, MD, who developed multiple sclerosis during medical school, was rebuffed from entering an internal medicine residency because of her disability. She was told, "Frankly, there are too many doctors in the country right now for us to worry about training handicapped physicians."[15] Dr Serena Young, an orthopedic surgeon who had polio as a child, experienced isolation and rejection during her residency.[16] The rejection she noted was not from her patients, but from her peers.

If the resident becomes disabled during training, this can create tremendous difficulties on many fronts. The other residents in the program may experience many conflicting emotions, including shock, commiseration for the colleague, feeling resentful that the call schedule will cause a greater burden on the other residents, and even the feeling of being threatened by facing the vulnerability of life. Because of these varied and diverse emotions, the other residents may be supportive, resentful, or distant in their relationships with their newly disabled colleague. As the physician-in-training with new limitations is trying to handle the immediate issues of managing new physical disabilities and learning new coping strategies, support—or lack of it—from supervisors and peers can have critical consequences.

After a period of convalescence, an individual may regain the ability to perform essential duties, while still requiring some minor modifications in the manner in which tasks are executed. It is not uncommon for residents to treat their colleague differently regardless of the individual's ability to perform. A flawed assumption may be made that the disability will render the resident incapable of returning to the program because of perceived insurmountable limitations. During this time, the returning resident may be quite concerned about the capacity to catch up, making support from colleagues and supervisors essential. Program directors and attending physicians should develop a strategy of positive reinforcement and support for the resident with physical challenges. The other residents are more likely to follow this positive example and also be supportive.

If the disability is so severe that return to residency is not possible, support for the resident by colleagues and supervisors is essential in maintaining a sense of identity and self-esteem that is so intimately intertwined with medical practice activities. Other outlets for the physician's resources should be explored so as not to let talent and knowledge go to waste.

Acquired Disabilities after Completion of Training

Some disabilities occur suddenly, for example, accidents, tumors, or complications from surgical procedures. In these cases, the physician has not had the opportunity to adjust life activities; day-to-day functioning may be a monumental struggle. Medical practice, which had previously played such a prominent role in life, is now relegated to the background as the immediate need for developing coping strategies for living takes precedence. Gradually, as the physician improves in function and in coping, medical practice may again feature prominently.

Colleagues who have witnessed the severity of the disability frequently have difficulty accepting the improvements, which have been so valiantly accomplished. In failing to acknowledge regained abilities, attempts to limit or restrict the clinician's activities are commonly encountered. This can be devastating for the physician, as identity is intimately intertwined with active practice. Support from family members and colleagues can be critical in overcoming these prejudicial attitudes. However, sometimes these attitudes cannot be changed and need to be avoided in order for the practitioner to succeed.[17] The attitude of colleagues may be a reflection of societal attitudes or perceived personal vulnerabilities.

Disabilities can sometimes be sudden and dramatic. For example, if a surgeon becomes quadriplegic after a car accident, performing surgery will clearly not be possible. However, contributions can still be made to a field by educating others through teaching or publishing, allowing valuable experience to continue to be shared, although in a different way. When the disability occurs early enough in the career path, a physician may choose to change specialties to a field that focuses more on primary care, psychiatry, radiology, pathology, or administration. Clearly, the education and experiences of physicians are precious resources that can be utilized in many ways.[18] Physicians who gradually acquire a disability may initially ignore its impact on their lives and medical practices. But as disorders progress, many emotions can develop: the physicians' fear of being unable to continue to practice, self-doubt after realizing their lives and medical practices may be permanently altered, or apprehensions about their colleagues' continued acceptance. As these changes are occurring, the physician can begin to develop techniques that will allow the continuation of medical practice.

The assistance of colleagues in developing these adaptations would be helpful but is rarely available. Thus, as the practitioner is attempting to develop new practice modalities, any missteps along the way might be erroneously viewed as evidence of lack of competence rather than a need for guidance.[19] Colleagues who can be trusted to be supportive and nonjudgmental can also help in identifying these adaptations. This is a critical factor, as some peers may automatically label the physician who is asking for assistance as one who is incapable of continuing an active practice. Therefore, it is important for the physician to seek out the correct colleagues from whom to gain support. This network is essential because inevitably there will emerge clinicians who challenge the professional with a disability. The capabilities of the disabled professional may be in question, and restrictions could be unjustly placed on his or her activities instead of identifying ways in which practice activities can continue. If one is lucky, a powerful mentor/advocate steps in to support and help the practitioner. For example, DeWitt Stetten, MD, developed visual impairment after being in active practice for many years. His support and strategies for coping came not from his colleagues or peers, but from other sources not associated with medical practice.

If employers or supervisors are approached to provide accommodations, this request should be viewed as between colleagues to avoid placing the requesting physician in a child-like, inferior position. The need for accommodations should be accepted gracefully, and all attempts to make the accommodation work properly should be made. It must be recognized that it is possible that initial attempts to provide accommodations may be insufficient or unsuitable. When this occurs, further or different accommodations may be required. Individuals who are not familiar with the needs of the disabled may make the erroneous assumptions that the clinician with physical challenges is hard to please and will never be satisfied. A more productive and positive approach would be to sit down with the physician to determine in what ways the accommodations could be modified to maximize the clinician's productivity.

Age-related disabilities may be particularly difficult for established physicians to handle. As people age, diabetes, cardiovascular disease, cerebrovascular accidents, Parkinson's disease, and chronic diseases can affect anyone, including physicians. These disorders may lead to fatigue, peripheral neuropathies, hemiplegia, and even cognitive difficulties. Age-related disabilities may be particularly challenging for the physician who has been in practice for many years, having gained respect and a reputation in the community. This can create a strong challenge to self-esteem and self-image, as the successful clinician's identity is often linked to professional accomplishments.

Professional colleagues who are also aging may be feeling threatened too and choose to restrict contact with the clinician as function deteriorates, feeling personally frightened of age-related disabilities.

Alternatively, they can be supportive, recognizing that these conditions can happen to anyone. Younger colleagues and partners may be too quick to write off the older clinician with a disability, negating continued abilities to contribute in useful ways, including active practice. Rehabilitation medicine and adaptive technology have enabled many individuals with disabilities to overcome their challenges and reenter the work force, leading full and active professional lives. An example of this was a primary care practitioner who experienced increased difficulty maintaining his practice because of progressive diabetes, peripheral neuropathies, and retinopathies. However, his patients of many years wanted to continue to see him because they had developed trust in his medical judgment.[20]

Psychosocial Factors

Many patients are quicker to accept the competence of a physician with a disability than are their professional peers. The natural rapport between physician and patient is eased by compassion, patience, creativity, and flexibility. The disabled physician has had to cultivate all these qualities while dealing with physical limitations.

Because the disabled are accustomed to working with others to accomplish tasks that cannot be completed independently, it is natural for clinicians with disabilities to acknowledge and respect the assistance provided by ancillary personnel. Patients may also feel less threatened by a physician who has shared with them the experience of undergoing medical treatment. Thus, their need to seek medical care is both validated and reinforced. When the clinician with a disability says, "I can understand what you are going through" to a person with a chronic medical condition, the patient realizes that these are not empty words. This promotes a genuine bond of trust between doctor and patient.

Psychosocial factors can impact greatly on the lives of physicians with altered abilities. It is essential for prospective physicians, even in the premedical curriculum, to associate and work with people with disabilities. Through professional interaction, they learn that a disability is not necessarily an illness, but it may make an individual different. The standard medical model teaches clinicians that *different* is equal to *illness* and must be fixed or cured. This misconception leads to difficulties in integrating the disabled into the general community, especially as equal members of the health care team. It may be hard for the able-bodied members of the medical community to accept the idea that the physician who has a disability may be completely and totally functional and independent, not needing to be "cured" to be effective. When we accept people with disabilities as part of our society, we will be better able to accept our colleagues with different abilities and help them to maximize their capabilities to contribute fully in the medical sciences. This may require different ways of executing tasks, different practice patterns, different modes of communication, and different ways of caring for patients. Although these methods are not considered mainstream medical practice, they are no less legitimate and are viable and safe ways to deliver competent medical care. Acknowledgment of the validity of difference can help all medical colleagues to treat each other equally, with respect and acceptance.

Thanks for coordination of this chapter to Joan Goddard, administrative assistant, JFK Johnson Rehabilitation Institute, Edison, New Jersey.

References

1. Tringo J. The hierarchy of preference toward disability groups. *J Spec Educ* 1970;4:295-306.

2. Moore-West MN, Heath D. The physically handicapped medical student in medical school: a preliminary study. *J Med Educ* 1982;57:918-921.

3.. Max W Rice DP, Trupin L. *Medical Expenditures for People with Disabilities.* Disability Statistics Abstract. 12. San Francisco: Disability Statistics Rehabilitation Research and Training Center, University of California; March 1996: 1-4.

4. Lewis SB. The physically handicapped physician In: Callan JP. *The Physician: A Professional under Stress.* East Norwalk, Connecticut: Appleton-Century-Crofts; 1983:318-326.

5. Martini CJM. Physical disabilities and the study and practice of medicine. *JAMA.* 1987;257:2956-2957.

6. Wainapel SW. Physical disability among physicians: an analysis of 259 cases. *Int Disabil Stud.* 1987;9:138-139.

7. Wainapel SW. The physically disabled physician. *JAMA.* 1987;257:2935-2938.

8. Read MR. Editorial comment: the disabled physician. *J Clin Psychiatry.* 1981;42:93.

9. Wainapel SW. The physician with a physical disability: the view from America. *Bull Assoc Disabled Professionals.* December 1983.

10. Struthers MS, Raphan M. The impact of the Americans with Disabilities Act on medical licensing and credentialing. *Med Law Pract.* 1997;80:47-49.

11. Nowlan D. Disabled doctors. *Irish Med J.* 1981;74:3.

12. Carrell S. Rejection by peers issue for handicapped MDS. *Am Med News.* July 1-8, 1983: 37-38.

13. Corbet B, Madorsky JG. Physicians with disabilities. *West J Med.* 1991;154:14-21.

14. Wainapel SW, Bernbaum M. Rehabilitation of the patient with visual impairment, in DeLisa JA, Ganz BM, Bockneck WL, et al, eds. *Rehabilitation Medicine: Principle and Practice.* 3rd ed. Philadelphia: WB Saunders Co; 1998:1733-1748.

15. Iezzoni LI. What should I say? *Harvard Med Alum Bull.* 1998;71:21-27.

16. LeBourdais E. Disabilities give some physicians a fresh insight into their profession. *Can Med Assoc J.* 1995;152:1492-1494.

17. Corbet B, Madorsky JG. Wounded healers. *New Mobility.* 1995;57:35-39.

18. Stelmach P. Handicapped physicians (letter). *Ann Intern Med.* 1985;102:271-272.

19. Moore DL. When bad things happen to good doctors: how physical disabilities affect medical career choices. Proceedings of the American Medical Women's Association 75th National Meeting, Philadelphia, November 4, 1990.

20. Wainapel SF, Bernbaum M. The physician with visual impairment or blindness. *Arch Ophthalmol* 1986;104:498-502.

Chapter 4

Physician Temperament, Psychology, and Stress

Malkah T. Notman, MD

Obviously, not all physicians are alike. With increasing emphasis on diversity in recruitment, variation is even more present than it was a generation ago. Medicine has also changed. The major technologic and information changes have affected diagnosis, treatment, and the skills necessary for both. The economic changes have meant that some of the personality traits that were adaptive a decade ago may now be problematic, such as a wish for autonomy in decisions and practice. Medicine has changed from being a male-dominated profession as far as numbers of physicians are concerned, and some entering medical school classes are more than half women. However, the models are still predominantly male in many aspects. This means that the conditions of training and work are still set up with expectations that work is dominant in the lives of physicians and students. Family needs and interests are seen as secondary. This varies to some extent with the specialty and with work conditions, such as hospital practice, HMOs, or office practice.

Medicine as a profession has consistently selected for certain types of personality. Women entering the field do create some differences, since the range of personality styles for women is somewhat different. However, there are some common characteristics that are important to recognize. In this chapter I will discuss these personality elements, the particular stresses of the training years, current stresses for physicians in practice, and some of the particular issues for women in medicine.

Characteristics of Physicians

People choose to be physicians for a variety of reasons. Interest in science, wishes to be useful and perform service or to "help people," or the influence of a childhood illness or illness in a family member can be important, as can a family doctor who was a hero or a mentor. Status, prestige, wishes for achievement, or even seeing medicine as a way of organizing one's life, if other goals seem vague, can be motivating. Less conscious influences can be the wish to know about the "secrets" of the body, or to learn the "inside" about people's lives. While the need to memorize and master a great deal of information has been lessened by new technology, a certain level of intellectual ability and drive *is* needed—and the capacity to reason and think quickly is a necessary baseline. Drive is necessary to sustain a student through medical training and also to make possible the long hours that are demanded.

Perfectionism and an organizational capacity can shade into a compulsive need to master and control and an obsessional style. Intellectual and obsessional defenses are also supported by the structure of medical training. The anxiety about knowing what to do and coping with responsibility tends to intensify compulsiveness. Perfectionism can also lead one to make higher demands of oneself and therefore to a greater possibility of a sense of failure. This can sometimes result in depression at being unable to meet one's goals and ideals.

Sometimes this orientation means that social relationships and connections are sacrificed in favor of work. This can lead to varying amounts of stress, particularly for women, for whom relationships are more commonly an important source of support and identity. The isolation that often accompanies medical training can be particularly stressful. This can continue for many years, not only during school but also during residency and often the early period afterward.

The need for control can also support a workaholic pattern. Doctors classically make poor patients because their need to be competent, active, and in a position of autonomy interferes with the need to be compliant as a patient and take direction and help from others. Denial has been described as a common problem for physicians, particularly when it concerns their own vulnerability or illness. Illness also threatens the work orientation on which self-esteem depends. It is difficult for physicians to tolerate feeling helpless. The ideal physician has often been portrayed as someone who is strong and can give help, provide answers, and give solutions. This is important in his or her self-image. It is a set of expectations that the patient brings to a relationship with a physician. Since the patient wants and expects help, the doctor is then endowed with power. Situations or people who create feelings of helplessness can make most physicians anxious. These patients or problems are then avoided. Thus, physicians are selected for those qualities of mastery and activity that make any situation of insecurity and dependency difficult. They also tend to avoid patients who have difficult personalities, have hopeless conditions, or are dying.

Tolerating a patient's emotion can be stressful for many physicians. A number of defense mechanisms are used to deal with this. One of these is objectifying the situation, that is, turning an illness and a suffering human being into a problem. This creates some distance and helps the physician to think actively and not feel personally involved, with its attendant risk of getting burned out because of the emotional strain. The black humor that is often described as being seen among physicians, such as joking about death, also establishes distance and the illusion of mastery. Yet the personal price paid can be considerable. The doctor can be seen as impersonal, lacking empathy, and appearing to ignore the emotional concerns of patients because of the limited focus on the "medical" problems.

Another personality style of dealing with the constant emotional demands of a practice is to avoid affect in many situations. For some physicians, this means avoiding spending a lot of time with one's own family as well and trying to ignore the stress this puts on familial relationships. Women physicians have been described as being less likely to do this, and it may be a source of chronic tension within the physician's family. Dividing up household responsibilities and making arrangements for child care and other responsibilities still leave the job of dealing with aggression and other difficulties with the children. With the increase in women physicians, a number of new patterns have developed. For some families there is sharing of child care, but often the woman remains the organizer and responsible "CEO" of the family.

Stresses on Physicians

The status and social position of the physician have changed in the past two decades from one of universal esteem to one that is attacked from many quarters. The challenges to the doctor's authority, for example from managed care and regulatory organizations, are a source of frustration and an interference with patient care. These challenges can also touch on important personality characteristics and can produce embarrassment and shame as dependency and vulnerability are exposed, directly undermining the cornerstones of physicians' self-esteem.

Medical education shares many characteristics with other professional training and graduate schools. However some specific components are unique to medicine. The training is long and rigid, and usually there is an intensity of demands from the beginning that is unparalleled in other graduate or professional programs. Most training programs are also quite inflexible, and it is difficult to integrate personal needs with work demands. The training years also occur during the time when young adults usually are forming attachments (such as getting married or forming long-term intimate relationships) or making other kinds of commitments.

Most medical students and physicians marry. The demands of training and practice combined with other needs have been variously reported as leading to higher divorce rates. This is difficult to assess in the context of the current changes in family patterns with high divorce rates in the general population, where many dual-career families nonetheless make creative adaptations and do well. However, those students and physicians who want to combine family commitments and medical training, whether they are male or female, find that the institutions are often not set up to accommodate anything but the work demands, although nominally this has been changing. It may be particularly difficult for young physicians and those in training to deal with family pressures or peer pressures from friends and other people who are free to do other kinds of things in their lives. With the shift from solo and small practice to "jobs" with HMOs, groups, or other organizational patterns, it has become more possible to work specified and more limited hours. The consequent changes in career satisfaction and career development are yet to be assessed.

Stress and impairment have been frequently linked, and a wide variety of problems and symptoms have been attributed to stress. This rings true intuitively, but the concept of stress may be shorthand for a range of different factors. Stress is a difficult concept to define and to measure. The stress of competition, for example, can be experienced as positive and motivating, not only as difficult. The evidence of the connection between stress and impairment by itself is not conclusive. Isolation, for example, is a source of stress, but this is a different stress than the problems induced by crowding, and also different than time pressures. In turn, time pressures for a perfectionistic person with high, rigid standards can be more intense than for someone who is more casual and flexible. Some stresses can lead to gratifications in mastery, while others are eroding.

Most studies of stress in students, residents, and physicians indicate that, although all three groups can report high stress levels, stress does not by itself result in symptoms. A study comparing stress and depression in medical, law, and graduate students at one university did not find that medical students were more stressed but did find that women scored higher on scales indicating depressed mood than the men did. This is consistent with the general population, where depression is more prevalent in women.

The relationships between stress and impairment and also between stress and marital problems are unclear. Work and family stress have been linked with impairment. Most studies of stress in students, residents, and physicians indicate that, although stress is reported high for all of these groups, most is handled without evidence of impairment. The time demands, lack of support, and conflicting responsibilities do produce symptoms. In many medical settings, women have fewer support systems than men do. Single women residents are reported as being more at risk for symptoms than any other group.

Special Issues for Women Physicians

In the past, many issues for women physicians were related to their minority status. Isolation, feeling scrutinized, feeling that the one or two women in a particular position represented all womankind, and feeling and being excluded from the decision making or "the loop" have lessened. However, these issues are still a problem in upper-level management and academic positions and in situations regarding advancement and promotion. A much wider range of styles and behavior still is tolerated for men than women. Women in some positions in academic medicine and research still say they feel disloyal or guilty or regarded as not serious if they become pregnant and have a family. These attitudes can exist even though others in the same community do not experience them. They can operate subtly and not necessarily consciously.

Women now in midlife and midcareer are entering their peak practice years and may also be at the midlife point in their marriages. They grew up and were trained in an era when it required a high level of interest and conviction for a woman to enter a field where prevailing patterns of training, expectations, and practice had been set by men. The choice exposed them to questions about their "femininity." For some of these women, this was experienced as a challenge and a stimulus to competition; others continued to feel marginal.

Women were unwelcome in some settings, not treated as equal, and symbolically or actually not given their own "space" as colleagues. There were minor problems, such as the lack of changing rooms or on-call rooms for women in hospitals, and more serious ones, such as a limited choice of residency programs and opportunities for practice. How many group practices are specifying that a woman should be on the staff?

Self-esteem problems and depression are more prevalent in women than men in the population at large. Women physicians are no different in their vulnerability to these problems, in spite of being high achievers. When sexism exists, it reinforces problems in self-esteem as well as creating rage and feelings of helplessness. Having "special needs" such as family responsibilities or child care can also be embarrassing if the prevailing work patterns do not involve bringing up anything considered personal.

Women medical students are fundamentally similar to other women, although very high in achievement, competence, and work orientation. They do share with other women some well-studied personality features: a tendency to be more affiliative than men and more ready to express emotion, acknowledge distress and physical symptoms, and use health care facilities. They are responsive to the opinions of others, they tend to see things in context, and they tend to negotiate and seek compromises. Gilligan has described the differences in moral reasoning. Women view moral development as involving the understanding of responsibility and relationships. Men, on the other hand, see moral development as related to fairness and the understanding of rights and rules.

The traditionally "feminine" gender role was incompatible with the qualities formerly considered important in the selection of students for medicine. There is also a gender difference in the balance between nurturing and achievement wishes. Medicine has allowed men to express the need to provide caretaking and nurturance, without diminishing achievement needs or compromising what were considered "masculine" goals. The situation has been different for women. Nurturant qualities have been considered "feminine," but medicine has been seen in the past as an achievement-oriented and therefore "masculine" field. Thus, women have recurrent conflicts between achievement and nurturing goals. An additional barrier has been the need for a science background to study medicine. Until recently, this was less likely for women to choose.

The assertiveness, competitiveness, and independence that are supported in men run counter to traditional feminine values and the socialization of women. There are important gender differences in the development of aggression and independence. The developmental process in women clearly exerts a profound effect on aggression, assertiveness, competence, and mastery. Girls identify with their mothers, who have often internalized ideals of service and "doing for" others. For many years, medicine has been one way for a woman to attain high achievement and recognition and at the same time fulfill feminine values of care and nurturance.

The defense against sadism described by Gabbard and Menninger is more pervasive in women. The prohibitions against direct expression of aggression are more consistently part of feminine style. Awareness of being aggressive makes both men and women feel guilty and lose self-esteem. But an openly aggressive woman is also in conflict with an additional part of her ego ideal, that of femininity.

Both men and women physicians share the compulsive triad of doubt, guilt feelings, and an exaggerated sense of responsibility, as well as the tendency to employ reaction formation as a defense against aggression. However, women physicians are different in some important ways. They value intimacy and attachments more and are more vulnerable to their loss; they are more expressive; they also tend more toward conformity.

Women medical students and physicians may project or externalize their conflicts about activity and aggression, paying more attention to the criticisms—such as of superiors, colleagues, family—than to their own inner feelings. These conflicts can interfere with medical performance and also affect the choice of specialty and practice setting. Women are usually the accommodators who are sensitive to the opinions of others. A woman is not only more sensitive to the feelings of rejection and "dependency" but often more open about these feelings than a man might be, giving a false impression of insecurity and lack of knowledge. Concerns about separation can lead to guilt and loss of confidence. When the woman physician must choose between caring for a patient, being with her family, and tending to her own needs, she may see herself as neglectful or unable to give adequate care rather than simply making choices.

Women are often more expressive of feelings than men and therefore are more likely to report symptoms and distress. They are also more ready than men to consider seeking help and less likely to see this as incompatible with strength and competence. This may also make them appear more vulnerable than they are.

Intellectual and obsessional defenses are supported by medical training, as Gabbard and Menninger describe. These defenses are more prevalent in men and consistent with male personality styles. Women physicians need closeness more and feel stressed if time pressures interfere with relationships. Women are not so fully sustained as men by the approval of mentors or the pursuit of perfection. They too want mastery and want to serve and rescue others, but the isolation of work undermines a particularly vital part of life for them by impairing self-esteem and nurturance prohibited by professional relationships.

For women who are raised to be collaborative and adaptive and to make compromises, there may be conflict between these traits and their own ambitions and aggression. The role of caretaker of patients, families, and parents can be in opposition to wishes for success and advancement; these are less ambivalently supported for men. For some younger women, it is easier to express and act on their commitment to research, their wishes for success, and their competitive feelings than it has been for women in earlier generations. They feel less guilty about these, having grown up in an era where more traditional ideas of femininity are not so dominant. However, this is also uneven and varies with the part of the country and in different cultural groups.

A counterdependent style, that is, having to be competent in every situation, interferes with getting help or mentoring. This is true for both men and women, who each have different psychological vulnerabilities. For the man, "weakness" challenges his ideas of masculinity. For the woman struggling in a field in which she feels she must adopt a strong or even masculine style, "weakness" can make her feel unqualified and that she doesn't belong.

Pregnancy and Relationship Issues

The overlapping of the period of career building and the reproductive years creates dilemmas. There are different solutions, but the child care and work issues are almost universal in dual-career families. Traditionally, mothers are blamed for all that goes wrong. The anxieties created by the recent case of the nanny who was implicated in the death of an infant in Boston were accompanied by much criticism of the mother, a physician, who was working at the time. In addition, pregnancy provides special stresses.

Pregnancy is an intrusion of the personal life of the physician into the work situation, both because it is impossible not to notice it and because it affects work commitments. Although different work situations cope with this in different ways, there are often conflicts in time demands, loyalties, and concerns about the doctor's own health as compared to the needs of her patients.

Pregnancy also stirs up strong emotions both in patients and colleagues. It can evoke envy, competitiveness, both with the baby and the doctor, unresolved feelings about siblings (both of the patients and of the doctors), and anger. After the baby is born, the child care arrangements must be solved, but there may also be problems in balancing the emotional commitments.

Women physicians are usually married to physicians or high-achieving men. There can be problems in the timing of careers. The woman can be interested in developing her practice after children are older, when the man is already established, creating tensions about household responsibilities and child care.

The egalitarian relationships that exist during training or early marriage are often strained with the arrival of children. Long work hours and stress of the profession have been blamed for troubled marriages. Not all of the data actually bears this out. The most salient factor associated with subjective rating of marital adjustment of profession-als is the perceived level of emotional support for career pursuits given to oneself and one's spouse.

Traditionally, the wives of male physicians have found gratification in the husband's fulfillment and also in the role this provides for them. The husbands of women physicians are less rewarded in this role.

In one study, spouses of physicians complained about their spouses' fatigue, lack of available time, and the necessity to postpone gratifica-tion. The husbands felt overburdened by domestic responsibilities and conflicted by their wives' career demands. The wives of male physicians, even when they were sacrificing their own time and inter-ests in the past, were gaining status and fitting into traditional roles. With opening up of opportunities for women, the gratifications of the traditional roles were no longer the only ones possible.

Husbands of women physicians can feel that "on-call" demands of the wives are infringements on their own autonomy. For some couples, for example, the wife covers domestic responsibilities when her husband is on call, but when she is on call, the husband does not feel he can take over and she needs to get coverage at home.

The different patterns of relationships that tend to be characteristic for men and women also often make it difficult for a woman doctor to leave her patients. This may result in conflict as to whose patients can be left. Many women physicians thus can find themselves in the super-mom, super-physician position. Feeling the pressures to do everything gives them no personal time or space. Some can feel guilty at giving their own needs or wishes priority. The time and energy given to work can also help deal with inner dissatisfaction or disap-pointment. It provides justification since taking care of someone else is always "noble."

Conflicts of this sort can lead to unconscious undermining of success, particularly for women. Family needs, such as illness in parents or in-laws, introduce complications. It is rarely the man who takes on this responsibility. Not marrying has become a more acceptable lifestyle, as have gay and lesbian partnerships. However the single person living alone can pay the price in loneliness.

The changing health care delivery system has produced dilemmas. There have been more opportunities for a limited practice, which is an advantage for women with small children. However, there are also pressures for greater "productivity" measured in number of patients seen. These pressures result in poorer care and less role for the physician in determining care. Many physicians are leaving, retiring, and going on disability. Hospital mergers and closings have threatened and, in some cases, destroyed income, training, jobs, expectations, and life plans. The high costs of medical school debts create anxiety. It is reported that many women graduates have greater debts than men. Many women physicians have difficulty repaying their school debts and keeping up with malpractice premiums.

Conclusion: Management of Stress

Physicians often are so committed to work that they do not allow sufficient time for leisure. Work gratifies so many needs, to feel important, to be needed, to deal with feelings of helplessness or depression, that for some it is difficult to not work without feeling anxiety. Some schedule "relaxation" by active sports such as running. Nevertheless it is important to provide support for taking time for oneself and for family. Support by peers can ameliorate feelings of guilt and selfishness. The work demands and time away from home are a major source of marital and family discord.

Opportunities for identifying problems, communicating with others about them, and expressing feelings as well as developing action plans can be very important in reducing feelings of helplessness and discouragement. In some of the recent hospital mergers and closings, many physicians felt threatened, helpless, and hopeless. Leadership that provided a means to share these reactions with others and create ideas for action and change was enormously helpful.

Equating having difficulties with weakness makes expressing these difficult. Unstigmatized pathways and access to support systems can be very beneficial.

Suggested Readings

Cartwright L. Personality differences in male and female medical students. *Psychiatry Med.* 1972;3:213-218.

Epstein C. Encountering the male establishment: sex-status limits on women's careers in the professions. *Am J Sociol.* 1975;15:6-9.

Gabbard G. The role of compulsiveness in the normal physician. *JAMA.* 1985;254:2926-2929.

Gabbard G, and Menninger R. The psychology of the physician. In: Gabbard G, Menninger R, *Medical Marriage.* Washington, DC: APA Press; 1998: chap 3.

Gabbard G, Menninger R, and Coyne L. The time of our lives: sources of conflict in the medical marriage. In Gabbard G, and Menninger R, eds. *Medical Marriage.* Washington, DC: APA Press; 1988:11-22

Gilligan C. In a Different Voice. Cambridge, Mass: Harvard University Press; 1982.

Helmers KF, Danoff D, Steinert Y, et al. Stress and depressed mood in medical students, law students, and graduate students. *Academic Medicine.* McGill University; 1997;72(8):707-714.

Nadelson C, Notman M. What is different for women physicians? In: Schrieber S, Doyle B, eds. *The Impaired Physician.* New York: Plenum Press; 1983:11-25

Notman M, Nadelson C. Medicine: a career conflict in women. *Am J Psychiatry.* 1973;130:1123-1127.

Notman M, Nadelson C. Psychological issues for the woman physician. In: Gabbard G, Menninger R, eds. *Medical Marriage.* Washington, DC: APA Press; 1978:67-78.

Schrieber S. Emotional problems of physicians. In: Schreiber S, Doyle B, eds. *The Impaired Physician.* New York: Plenum Press; 1983:3-10.

Chapter 5

Physicians and Intimate Relationships

Michael Myers, MD

Mythology abounds about the health of intimate relationships of physicians, whether they be marriages, same-sex relationships, or unmarried cohabiting or separate living relationships. In fact, there are no recent empiric data on physicians' intimate relationships; old studies were largely of male physicians with traditional marriages. The divorce rate of physicians is apparently no higher than that of other groups of professionals. Female physician divorces are as prevalent as those of other female professionals, and virtually nothing statistically is known about the viability of lesbian and gay male physician relationships. However, there is much anecdotal evidence that physicians have their share of relationship challenges, joys, and heartaches.

Common Issues

Overwork as a Cause of Relationship Strain

A classic complaint in medical relationships is that the physician partner works too hard. This complaint embodies many charges:

- long working days at the office and/or hospital (leaving early in the morning and/or returning after family mealtime in the evening)
- frequent on-call responsibilities
- hospital rounds on weekends or deliveries that interrupt family life

- time taken up with other medically related activities, such as committees, meetings, and continuing education
- for physicians in academic medicine, time devoted to research, presenting papers at medical meetings, writing grant proposals, writing articles for publication, teaching medical students and residents, and some clinical practice

All physicians in relationships who are accused by their partner of overworking need to ask themselves how much their commitment to work is self-serving. Physicians should consider the following questions:

- Am I asking more of my partner and my children than I should?
- Would most partners of someone working as hard as I am feel short-changed?
- Am I more interested in pleasing my patients and in professional advancement than in devoting time to my partner and his/her needs?
- Could I be more efficient and organized at work and still be a good physician?
- Do I need to say "no" to patient, student, colleague, and employer demands on my time so I can be at home more?

Case vignette. Dr A, a neurosurgeon, and his wife, Dr B, a pathologist, sought consultation when Dr B told her husband that the marriage was over. She argued that she was fed up with his long hours, his "fast track" academic commitments, his trips away to medical meetings to present scientific papers, and his exhaustion and self-centeredness when he was at home. Her loneliness contributed to her falling in love with a man at work, another pathologist. Unfortunately, there was little that could be done about their marriage at this late stage. Dr B left her husband. The devastated husband continued in individual therapy for support through the separation. Once he was feeling stronger, he was able to look at his work and how out of balance his life was. He left academic life, joined a group practice, worked fewer hours, and took up a number of new interests.

In many relationships today, it is not just physicians who are guilty of overwork. Indeed, overwork is very common in both partners in a relationship. This includes two-paycheck couples and single-earner relationships. Even some male physicians in traditional marriages complain that their wives are working harder than they are and "are never home," referring to their children's school and extracurricular activities and activities at houses of worship and in the community.

When couples are able to freely discuss their concerns about work, they can build understanding, make constructive changes, or at least make some short-term compromises with each other. If they can't, relationship symptoms will arise:

- communication breakdown
- bickering or arguing without resolution
- resentment
- fatigue
- loneliness and vulnerability to an extramarital affair
- distancing from each other
- sexual difficulties

Overwork as a Result of Relationship Strain

For most physicians, medicine is quite engaging, and there is usually plenty of it. Some physicians who work a lot are actually running away from problems at home that they can't see or don't see (ie, denial), that are too painful to face, or that they feel ill-equipped to solve. Examples include the following:

- Basic, bread-and-butter communication hurdles that all couples must confront
- Entrenched communication breakdown that has created a home atmosphere of formality, stiffness, and sterility, or its opposite, a highly charged, volatile, explosive, and possibly violent milieu
- Parental responsibilities, such as helping with the child or children, which can result in the physician having a very peripheral, nonintimate, and breadwinner relationship with the family

- Illness in one's partner or spouse such as cancer, HIV/AIDS, depression, or substance abuse

- A partner or spouse whom one no longer loves, but from whom separation or divorce is anathema to one or both partners

Case vignette. When Dr C, a rheumatologist, and Ms D, an attorney, came for help, they echoed each other's chief complaint: "Our lives are very busy so we don't have a lot of time for each other. When we do get together, all we do is fight. Can you help us communicate better?" Efforts and exhortations to each of them to work less and to schedule time together fell on deaf ears: something always came up, one would get sick, or one would "forget." They were not able to spend any time alone together until they worked in couples therapy on several unresolved issues they had swept under the carpet: Ms D's breast cancer five years earlier and her sense that her husband was not there for her; Dr C's daily use of marijuana and Ms D's displeasure with this; Ms D's "shopping compulsion" and Dr C's unexpressed rage at this; and their teenage daughter's boyfriend, whom Dr C couldn't stand because of his race and whom Ms D really liked. Dr C and Ms D coped by throwing themselves into their work, as had their dual-career parents when they were growing up.

Trouble Communicating

Obtaining a medical degree does not guarantee a facility or gift for intimate communication with a loved one. How to nurture and make a relationship flourish over the years is not taught in medical school. In fact, medical training and medical work may actually work against achieving and maintaining intimacy with a partner or spouse. Why?

- Rigorous medical study and exclusive devotion to work remain prevalent in most training programs, today with scant attention being paid to trainees' personal and relationship lives.

- The time demands expected of trainees and practicing physicians today are not in keeping with changing demographics, ie, most physicians do not have someone at home to do "everything," and partners and spouses are human too!

- Some of the best teachers, clinicians, and researchers lead very unbalanced lives and do not model for those of the next generation how to have intimacy at home. Indeed, some mock that, and those who do have successful intimate relationships rarely talk about this with their students or residents.

- How physicians communicate with their patients (where they are in charge and ideally balance clinical neutrality and professional compassion) is very different from intimate communication with a loved one (where they are often very vulnerable, naked, and not in charge).

Physicians' communication troubles with their partners or spouses are really no different from those of other couples. For example:

- Not making or protecting the time to talk to each other

- Talking about superficial or safe subjects only, thereby not taking risks with each other

- Talking without communicating, ie, they do not get their messages across to each other

- Talking that leads to tension, arguing, defensiveness, frustration, withdrawal, and exhaustion

- Talking that results in verbal or physical violence

It is wise to remember that intimate communication involves different levels of talk, including:

1. *Conscious and verbalized.* This is uncensored and uninhibited talk that flows smoothly and easily in both directions. Information is exchanged. It feels good, it's safe, and it's often energizing and restorative.

2. *Conscious and not verbalized.* There are some or many things that physicians are aware of but do not share because they may be simply private and not used to sharing. This may be characterologic. They may be embarrassed or guilty about certain issues. They may hold back because an earlier attempt to talk about these matters, or something similar, with the partner led to a fight, tears, defensiveness and counterattack, or shaming, and they

don't want to go there again! They may erroneously assume, in a mind-reading way, that the partner is going to have some kind of negative reply to what they have to say, so they don't say it.

3. *Unconscious and not verbalized.* This is beyond awareness. Physicians may get glimpses in their dreams, or if they have had too much to drink and lose their inhibitions and say things that they do not normally say to their partner. Sarcasm may be indicative of unconscious hostility. It behooves individuals to pay attention to these matters if they are puzzled by their communication blockages.

A word about gender and communication. It is not true that women communicate better than men. It is true that women tend to communicate differently from the way men do. Women tend to define themselves more in terms of relationships; hence, it is natural to have concerns about relationship health and functioning. Men value autonomy and independence. Not that relationships are not important to men in medicine, but they rarely understand how much their medical work impacts on their committed relationship. They may assume that their relationship is fine, they do not wish to be bothered about it, or they feel that if one's partner or spouse is unhappy, then it's that person's fault. Male physicians often find preventive talking about the relationship difficult, foreign, or boring. When they do come to accept that there is indeed a relationship problem, they are more reluctant to seek professional help and often feel guilty and embarrassed. Most referrals to a therapist still tend to be female-initiated in heterosexual couples.

Alcohol and Other Drug Use

The rates of alcohol and drug abuse and dependence in physicians and their partners are not diminishing, despite some innovative teaching programs in our medical schools and training programs, as well as earlier intervention and treatment. Excessive use of drugs, including alcohol, is a common complicating factor in physician relationships. Although relationship strain occasionally leads to use and overuse of alcohol, marijuana, and proprietary sedatives and sleeping pills, the problem is usually the other way around. Medical couples develop relationship symptoms and personal unhappiness because one of them has developed a chemical abuse or dependency pattern.

Both male and female physicians become addicted. Many in medicine have biological relatives with chemical dependency, which makes them at risk based on both genetic and psychosocial vulnerabilities. Alcohol, of course, is readily available to all citizens. But many physicians have access to pharmaceutical samples with abuse potential. Also, physicians generally are able to self-prescribe. Furthermore, some physicians prescribe habit-forming or addictive drugs to their physician-patients quite liberally or in a cavalier manner at variance with how they treat lay patients. In addition, the well-meaning physician may be manipulated by an addicted colleague into inappropriate prescribing.

For many reasons (denial, secretive use, minimization, shame, and fear of licensure reporting and investigation), it is usually the affected physician's partner or spouse who first labels this as impairing the relationship, wants to address it, and wants professional help. Although drug abuse in physician relationships is quite common, it is rare for a physician to present with a statement like, "I have developed a problem with alcohol and it's affecting my relationship. Can you help us?" It is impossible for many physicians to see their use of the drug as a problem, and if they do, it is difficult to admit that they need professional help unless things have really fallen apart and they have lost the relationship or it is in serious jeopardy.

Because this problem is so common in physician relationships, one should listen carefully and openly to any loved one who expresses concern about a physician's drug use. It is really rare for someone who loves a physician to be wrong about this subject or to be overreacting! Furthermore, all those who treat physicians and their partners should look for this as a causative or exacerbating factor in relationship dysharmony and to be sensitive and gentle yet firm in its uncovering. Chapter 8 discusses substance use disorders more fully.

Psychiatric Illnesses Other than Addictions

Physicians are probably not immune from any condition in the DSM-IV, the official diagnostic classification of mental diseases. Certain disorders, however, stand out because of their frequency among physicians and/or because of their effects on intimate relationships. They are:

- *Mood disorders* – depression (all types) and bipolar illness

- *Anxiety disorders* – which includes panic disorder, posttraumatic stress disorder, social and specific phobias, and obsessive-compulsive disorder. Mood and anxiety problems are discussed in more detail in Chapter 6.

- *Adjustment disorders* – a symptom complex that is related to an external stressor and is often characterized by anxiety or depressive symptoms, or a change in behavior (often noted in the physician's workplace by others)

- *Eating disorders* – more common in women in medicine, but also seen occasionally in male physicians

- *Cognitive impairment or psychiatric symptoms caused by a general medical condition* – alcohol or other drugs, metabolic impairment and delirious states, dementias, vascular disorders, demyelinating diseases, Parkinson's disease, head trauma, and HIV infection are some examples

- *Personality disorders* – such as borderline, narcissistic, or obsessive-compulsive type

There is an intricate relationship between personal mental health and intimate relationships; unfortunately, physicians who suffer from a psychiatric illness are more prone to relationship distress, conflict, and relationship breakdown. Also, because of assortative mating, it is not unusual for both members of a couple to have or be prone to psychiatric illnesses. This can make life together quite precarious; however, rarely are both partners ill at the same time, so that one of them will be stable when the other is unwell and can provide support and take over more responsibilities, both at home and perhaps in the workplace. It is hard to be a "good" partner or spouse when you don't feel well, when you're having panic attacks, when you're depressed, or if you're cognitively impaired. And it is hard to be a "good supporter" indefinitely because of fatigue from doing double duty and not getting sustenance in return.

Taking mood disorders as an example, some of the more common symptoms of depression are trouble concentrating, inability to listen for long, slowed thinking, distorted or obsessively focused thinking, suspiciousness, decreased energy, decreased interest in doing things, less or no interest in sex, irritability, poor sleeping, decreased appetite or overeating, increased dependency, and self-absorption. All of these symptoms affect intimate relationships, especially communication, connection, function, and closeness.

It helps when physicians and their partners can discuss how the illness has affected their relationship—the sadness that both partners may feel, the exhaustion and dispiritedness if the person has been ill for quite a while or is not responding very quickly to treatment, the loss of the good times that they used to have together, the erosion of closeness and sexual togetherness, and the fear, rational or not, that the relationship might end.

Case Vignette. Dr E and her husband were referred for couples therapy because they had decided to separate and the family physician thought they should have a trial of therapy. Dr E lived with bipolar illness and had just been discharged from the hospital after attempting suicide by taking an overdose of various medications. This was not a mutual decision to separate—in fact, neither of them wanted to separate, but Dr E thought that they should separate because she was "garbage" and a burden. On further questioning, it became clearer that Dr E was still very depressed, continued to feel suicidal, and was delusional in her self-perceptions of unlovableness and uselessness. She felt fraudulent as a pediatrician, wife, and mother. She was readmitted to the hospital, and she improved with ECT. Once she was well, the two of them responded nicely to a few supportive conjoint visits and a group for families living with a loved one with a mood disorder.

Sexual Concerns

Physicians are no more prone to sexual difficulties in their relationships than the general population. Sexual difficulties include:

- Disorders of sexual desire or interest
- Disorders of sexual arousal: erection difficulties in men and lubrication difficulties in women
- Disorders of orgasm: premature and retarded ejaculation in men and orgasmic inhibition in women
- Sexual orientation conflicts: concerns about bisexuality or homosexuality that may affect sexual intimacy
- Dyspareunia and/or vaginismus
- Gender identity disorder (identification with the opposite sex, which may include a wish or desire to live as the opposite sex)
- Paraphilias (eg, voyeurism, cross-dressing, exhibitionism)

Disorders of sexual desire in one or both partners are the most common sexual complaints in physician couples. Sometimes it is due to simple fatigue and the pressures of leading very busy lives, a well-known phenomenon today. However, sometimes feeling "too tired" masks an underlying tendency to channel most of one's sexual energy into work or sport. This may also represent a disguised problem with one's self-esteem or sense of attractiveness; an awkwardness, inexperience, rigidity, and naivete about sex; an undiagnosed mood disorder that causes diminished libido; or an unrecognized and unexpressed problem with relationship slights, put-downs, hurts, and resentments.

Although the key to addressing and overcoming most sexual concerns in relationships is communication, most couples do not easily talk about their sexual lives together. Physicians do not discuss sex any more easily than nonphysicians do. Any comfort or facility that they have with their own sexuality is almost always a reflection of their personal life experience, not what they have learned from lectures, textbooks, or clinical practice.

In many couples, each partner blames the other for a lack of sexual desire or for not initiating sex often enough. This can be very confusing, and gender also seems to play a role. Women admit more easily to a change or loss of interest in sex. Many male physicians seem to have difficulty admitting to themselves and to their partners their lack of interest in making love. They are sexually ready and enjoy having sex, but this may not be "making love" as defined by their female partner. Romantic gestures, spending time together talking, relaxing together, feeling loved and honored—essentials of making love—take time and energy and are very different from "having sex."

Common Problem Situations

Extrarelationship Affairs

The intimate relationships of physicians usually include a covenant and expectation of fidelity. Hence, unfaithfulness almost always poses a threat to the sanctity or strength of this bond and can upset relationship integrity and function. Most couples who are facing recent disclosure or knowledge of an outside relationship find themselves in crisis, and both the physician and his/her partner may feel quite symptomatic. Indeed, they may have an intensity of feeling (fright, panic, despondency, suspiciousness, embarrassment, rage, jealousy) or thought (paranoia, violence, retribution, homicide, suicide) that they have never before experienced.

What causes affairs to occur? There are reasons that center on the individual and those that implicate the relationship.

Individual Reasons. Reasons that primarily involve the individual include:

- Immaturity (being too young to commit to a relationship), a particularly common cause of an outside relationship in medical student and resident intimate relationships

- Inner conflict—for example, poor self-esteem is offset by attention from others

- Alcohol or other drug usage—produces disinhibition

- Depression or bipolar illness—depressed individuals are vulnerable to the excitement or interest of another; manic individuals feel sexy and lack caution

- Character defect—may lack conscience or guilt about sex with someone other than their chosen partner

- Sexual addiction/compulsive sexuality—repeated sexual gratification is sought out in a driven fashion

- Life-stage factors—an example is the male "menopause" at midlife

- Job threat or job loss—shattered self-esteem or unworthiness leads to vulnerability to the attention or affection of others

Relationship Reasons. Reasons that more involve the couple as a unit include:

- Boredom or loneliness

- Partner is "busy"—when physicians are preoccupied with their practices, being on call a lot, studying for examination, the loved one feels unloved

- Partner is sick—and unavailable to the loved one for companionship, conversation, sex, and so forth

- Pregnancy or postpartum stage—the male partner feels upstaged by the developing fetus or new baby

- Changed relationship sexuality—less frequent, less passionate, less mutual erotic satisfaction

- Diminished intimacy at home—less warmth, closeness, sharing, and laughter

- Miscellaneous—when one's partner has let himself/herself "go" (in appearance) or when one's partner has gotten "old"

Because outside relationships are best managed by prevention, all physicians should heed the warning signals that they might be heading toward an affair. They are:

- Not feeling loved or appreciated at home (this may or may not include a change in their sexual relationship)

- Brooding or feeling resentful about this and not talking about it

- Closing off from their partner and being more distant in time together, interests, and activities
- Having a feeling of not wanting to go home despite feeling tired after working all day
- Stopping off for a drink or two on the way home
- Noticing more than usual attractive and interesting individuals in one's everyday life
- Beginning to fantasize and/or dream about one or more of these people
- Feeling nervous or excited around these individuals
- Feeling tempted to act on these thoughts or feelings, or feeling vulnerable to individuals who express interest in them

Medical Illness in the Physician, Partner, or Child

For some physicians, developing a medical disorder, especially one that is chronic and debilitating (or has that potential), is extremely difficult psychologically. In addition to the feelings that beset all of humankind (shock, fear, anger, grieving, and so forth), there may also be guilt or shame. Such physicians blame themselves, feel that they are letting others down, feel inferior in the eyes of their peers, and often do not easily talk about their inner state. Why? Postulated reasons include an overdeveloped sense of perfectionism that allows for no flaw; a particularly harsh conscience that is rigid and punitive, and that may be projected onto others, eg, that colleagues are judging; a real or true perception that indeed their fellow physicians are uncaring and unempathic; mistrust of others who may gossip and breach confidentiality; and realistic fears that their job security and/or ability to practice medicine may be threatened, with serious and understandable financial implications. For these reasons, physicians living with illness can become morbidly egocentric and depressed, and this impacts on their intimate relationships.

Case Vignette. Dr and Mrs F came for marital therapy about 6 months after Dr F was diagnosed with ulcerative colitis. Mrs F started: "My husband's driving me nuts—you would think that he is the only person to ever have this diagnosis—he is obsessed with his diet, his bowel, his appetite, his weight, his energy, you name it. He won't eat in restaurants with me anymore. He won't go to Mexico because he's afraid of a bug. I'm going mad. His gastroenterologist is fed up with both of us and won't return my telephone calls. You know what—I don't blame him!" Dr F didn't deny that he was very worried—he had never been sick a day in his life, and he said that he felt very sad that their marriage had come to this. After the first visit, it was decided to treat Dr F individually. He really needed to talk about his fears of worsening bowel involvement, drug reactions, infections, colectomy, and ileostomy as well as his isolation about the disease, his embarrassment about rectal colonoscopy exams, and his fears of not being a good physician, provider, husband, and father. He and their marriage did very well.

What about medical illness in the physician's partner or spouse? This can threaten the relationship in different ways. Sometimes, physicians do not take seriously the ills of loved ones, so they may feel angry, disrespected, and abandoned. These feelings may compound the illness and worsen the physical symptoms, or the person becomes depressed or begins to drink too much or abuse prescribed painkillers and tranquilizers. This situation is most common when the physician is overworking, puts his/her profession ahead of everything else, and is out of touch with the relationship; the physician uses adaptive clinical armor (clinical neutrality and measured empathy) at home; the physician is overly perfectionistic and does not accept illness personally or in loved ones; or the partner is not forthright and direct in admitting and explaining the illness, pain, and so forth. This reluctance may define his/her personality, ie, hates to bother others, needs to be self-reliant, feels unworthy, or is depressed and can't articulate what is needed from others.

Sometimes, physicians have difficulty demarcating their role as a partner from their role as a physician. They may become overinvolved by interfering in or undermining the management of the physician who is treating their partner, by giving their partner medications themselves, or by yielding to the demands of their partner for medical care as opposed to simply being supportive. This may become very serious, and the partner ends up receiving inadequate and/or dangerous care, while their relationship changes from one of intimate partners to doctor-patient.

When it is the physician's child who is ill, some of the above dynamics may occur, and this leads to misunderstandings, tension, and flawed communication. Here are some possible reasons:

- Some physicians regularly and unabashedly treat their own children, to the chagrin of the primary care physician and pediatrician. If this is against the partner's wishes, this creates conflict.

- If delivering the care to the afflicted child is not balanced in some way, there can be exhaustion and resentment in the partner who is the primary caretaker. Therefore, even in traditional relationships wherein the physician is the sole wage earner, he or she should strive to do his/her share in the evenings and over weekends. This ensures good bonding and a healthy parent-child relationship—and helps to offset family misalignments, with mother and child being tightly and overemotionally involved with each other and the father being off on the sidelines.

- When or if the child is hospitalized and if the physician-partner does not visit outside of his/her regular working day, this reinforces a doctor-patient model more than a parent-child model. Even the treating physicians may relate to the physician more like a fellow physician or member of the "treatment team" rather than a concerned and possibly worried parent of a sick child. This can lead to distancing and affect closeness in the physician's relationship with his/her partner.

When the Physician Is Sued

The threat of being sued and the reality of a malpractice suit are part of practicing medicine today. Akin to this, and no less traumatic, is when physicians are investigated by their state licensing boards. How does this affect intimate relationships?

The symptoms or change in behavior that one can develop when in the midst of a lawsuit typically include:

- irritability
- despondency
- anxiety
- insomnia
- embarrassment
- frustration and bitterness
- loss of work satisfaction
- withdrawal from one's family and social activities
- emotional distancing from patients
- hypervigilance at work, eg, self-doubts, checking, and unnecessary tests
- premature retirement

Rarely are the physician's partner and other loved ones spared. The whole family may feel the stress, particularly if there is coverage in the media. Sometimes the entire family colludes in denying that anyone is feeling the effects, and if they do not speak about it outside the home, they may feel very isolated. In some communities, physicians and their partners are shunned by medical colleagues, and, if a preexisting psychiatric illness such as substance dependence contributed to the mishap, then there may be layers of personal and relationship distress. Immediate or urgent psychiatric consultation may be necessary, especially if there is a risk of suicide.

All sued physicians and their partners should be offered assistance because of the strain that this type of assault, often protracted, has on relationship harmony. Support groups can be very helpful—as can other physicians and their partners who have been through a lawsuit themselves getting together with the recently sued physician and his/her partner. Empathy and reassurance are key. Ventilation of feelings about the matter (not the case particulars) is healing and may need to be done multiple times.

Additional Issues for particular Types of Relationships

Interracial, Interethnic, and Interfaith Relationships

Given the cultural mosaic of our medical centers and the cosmopolitan nature of the cities where physicians most commonly live and practice, it is not unusual for doctors to form intimate relationships with someone of a different background. These relationships tend to be exciting and interesting; however, as commitment deepens and if marriage (or a commitment ceremony in same-sex relationships) and children are being considered, strain may break out because of a resurgence of feelings and ideas associated with family and cultural values. Even when couples themselves are not struggling with their differences, they may feel pushed and pulled by their respective families of origin, who express strong feelings about the relationship of their adult children. This then impacts on the couple, especially if those family members do not accept the relationship or refuse to attend a wedding of mixed faith.

Case Vignette. Mr G and Ms H, cohabiting medical students, came for help because they were fighting a lot, avoiding each other, and no longer making love. They had attributed most of their difficulties to their rigorous study, on-call schedules, and worry about exams. However, they wanted an opinion on whether the fact that both sets of parents were refusing to attend their proposed wedding might be significant. They were of different races and faiths. There had never been any intermarriage in either of their families. Both fathers were physicians on faculty of the local medical school. It was necessary to validate the isolation and family estrangement that these two were feeling and how that was impacting on their solidarity. The suggestion that they continue to talk and negotiate with their families over time was received well—as was a meeting with both sets of parents and the two of them. They were prepared by doing a series of role plays with them so that they could handle just about anything! They did get married—with lots of compromises, tears, and joy—and both families in attendance.

International medical graduates (IMGs) who marry someone of a very different background may experience even more stress. They may have problems with their visas and whether they can remain in the country. They may have worries about their families at home who want them to return, yet their new partner may have no desire to do so. Because some IMGs send money home to their families, this can cause strain in their intimate relationships and conflict around divided loyalties. Some IMGs encounter discrimination in North America and cannot always find work as easily as someone who is a graduate of a US medical school. His/her partner may not understand this or may resent it. Also, some IMGs struggle with acculturation, including mastering English, and this can affect their self-esteem. In highly competitive residencies or medical communities, if IMGs are having personal or relationship problems, they may be reluctant to seek professional help because "I can't show any chinks in my armor, I have to be twice as good as my American-educated colleagues." Further, they may come from a country wherein mental health care is even more stigmatized and misunderstood than in North America.

In smaller or rural communities, it may be hard for couples to find a therapist who is comfortable treating them and fully appreciates all of their issues. It is imperative that the therapist not only recognize his/her own differentness but also discuss race, ethnicity, and faith openly and with sensitivity and professionalism. Even seasoned and well-trained therapists can never fully appreciate the nuances, idiosyncrasies, and subtleties of values, roles, expectations, language, and speech in couples with unique and rich individual biographies.

Dual-doctor Couples

Couples in which both partners are physicians are really no different than other dual-career couples. Both individuals have similar levels of higher education and commitment to paid work outside the home. Both are defined, to a greater or lesser degree, by being a physician, although the magnitude or centrality of this is often greater in male physicians than female physicians. Dual-doctor couples tend to be egalitarian, with a mutual respect for each other's intelligence, calling, and commitment to family responsibilities. They rely on each other's income and each other's attitudes to sharing child care and household labor.

Some of the types of problems that can and do occur in two-physician couples include:

1. When the man views his career as more important than his partner's. He may not consider a geographical move if she is offered a fellowship or a promotion. If one of the children is ill or has a doctor's appointment, she has to cancel her patients. He supports maternity leave but not paternity leave. He puts down her branch of medicine as not being as important as his.

2. When, despite their both being physicians, one of them lacks understanding and/or empathy for the other's long working day, difficult patients, on-call demands, and interruptions of family life. In fact, it is often because the complaining partner is a physician that he/she can see that things are out of control, that their partner is burning out, disorganized, not delegating responsibility, and not functioning as efficiently as before.

3. When there has been a shift in power. This is most common when women physicians are practicing part-time and raising small children. Because she is at work fewer hours per week and is earning less money, she begins to feel "out of the loop" professionally and to feel less valued at home by her partner. Indeed, their relationship may now be skewed toward a traditional type of marriage where she is doing absolutely everything at home, ie, CEO of the home and all of the unpaid labor—and still seeing patients! Her partner is increasingly engaged with his career and doing less and less at home. This situation quickly leads to resentment, tension, misunderstandings, and unhappiness.

4. When their professional lives are so busy that their relationship suffers. This is most common in couples with children but also occurs in dual-doctor couples in very demanding branches of medicine or when they are both on an academic "fast track." Most of these couples find that they need to make a deliberate and continuing effort to preserve and protect time for each other.

Without this concerted attention, they run the risk of "waking up" years down the road to a complete stranger despite their achievements and family or couple veneer of "having it all."

5. When their relationship is as "professional" as their careers. In other words, they relate to each other as medical colleagues, roommates, or business partners. There is no problem if each of them thrives like this or is content; and there are many two-professional couples who do. Conflict, frustration, and relationship loneliness occur only if one wants or both of them want more intimacy, shared affection, sexuality, and so forth.

6. When there is a significant age difference between the two members of the couple, the most common being an older male physician and his younger female physician-partner. These relationships not uncommonly begin in hospital settings or other medical venues. Classically, the male physician is unhappily married or newly separated and begins a relationship with the female physician who is a medical student, resident, or young attending. If they met in a supervisor-supervisee setting, this makes things more complicated because of boundary issues, role blurring, and a power differential. What these couples need to watch for, anticipate, and be able to discuss are potential complications of life-stage differences (both personally and professionally): he stalls at leaving his wife or getting on with his divorce while she loathes being "the other woman" or fears simply "being dumped"; he is settled into what he is doing professionally and is immobile while she is in training or just beginning and would like to go elsewhere for a fellowship or new position; he has children plus a vasectomy while she would like kids of her own; he is somewhat controlling and often denying it, which she initially accepts, only to later rebel against it as she matures and becomes more confident in herself; he develops sexual insecurities and becomes jealous and possessive, which confuses and alarms her; he finds her somewhat naive and unexposed, which causes him to feel lonely and her to feel put down; he begins to develop health problems and she panics at being cast into a caretaker role both at work and at home: suddenly her partner has become "an old man."

Gay and Lesbian Physician Couples

Like most physicians, gay and lesbian doctors desire and strive for a close, loving relationship with one particular person, someone who is interested in both individual freedom and personal commitment. Gay and lesbian couples are more similar than different from heterosexual medical couples. They too have problems balancing work and family, overworking, communicating effectively, making love, coping with illness, and so forth. Despite major societal advancements in recognition of domestic partnerships (protection of assets and property rights, custody rights, health and pension benefits, and commitment ceremonies), these battles have been hard fought. Segments of society remain virulently antihomosexual, and this prevents some gay and lesbian physicians and their partners from living openly in their communities with acceptance and dignity. The psychological significance of this basic attitudinal difference toward gay and lesbian couples, as opposed to heterosexual couples, must not be underestimated. What are some of the unique concerns and problems of gay and lesbian physicians in intimate relationships?

Gay Male Couples. Some of the particular issues faced by couples composed of two men include:

1. *Competition.* Men are socialized to be independent, autonomous, strong, and competitive. Some branches of medicine thrive on competition. Common areas of competition are money, intelligence, success at work, sports, sexual prowess, physical attractiveness to other men, culinary skill, and taste in art and design. These are surface matters that may produce relationship tension, arguing, and distancing. However, these issues are often masking, in one or both of them, underlying problems with self-esteem, self-acceptance, trust, commitment, and security in the relationship.

2. *Sexual acting out.* Men tend to act out their difficulties with each other by having sex with other men rather than recognizing and talking about their unhappiness, slights, loneliness, and resentment. They are hurting and vulnerable and may find themselves "cruising" for sex with strangers, ie, "looking for love in all the wrong places" or actually falling in love with another man.

Case Vignette. Dr I and Dr J, both residents, presented in the midst of a huge relationship crisis. Dr I came home from work one day and confessed that he was having an affair with a medical student on his service. Dr J was horrified, not only because his relationship was in jeopardy but also because of the ethical issues associated with supervisor-trainee dynamics (although both Dr I and his student were trainees, Dr I was supervising the student and evaluating him for the program director). There were lots of reasons why their relationship was strained and Dr I was vulnerable: they were a closeted couple (Dr I was in orthopedics and Dr J in urology), so they had few external supports; they each were on call a lot and could not always coordinate their schedules; although they had a good sexual relationship, neither communicated feelings of love, tenderness, vulnerability, or insecurity very easily; and Dr I was on probation, which made him feel very second-rate and ashamed, yet he never shared these feelings with Dr J. After two conjoint visits to get these two men talking to each other again with more honesty and mutual sensitivity than ever before, Dr I ended the relationship with his student. This young man, fortunately and with grace, accepted this decision with no fallout at work or reporting to the program director.

3. *Intimacy struggles.* Accepting love from and giving love to another man may be a dance, a push-pull dilemma. Many gay men acknowledge their comfort and ease with sex but their discomfort and difficulty with connection, depth of feeling for another, and commitment. They may erroneously associate a committed relationship with dependence and entrapment, not seeing that a healthy relationship has a balance of autonomy and intimacy. Unless they can communicate their feelings verbally to some degree, their sexual relationship will get bogged down, suffering in frequency, emotional intensity, and satisfaction.

4. *"Coming out" disparities.* Couples can experience strain when one of them is far along in his acceptance of his homosexuality and its disclosure to family and close friends, while his partner is quite ambivalent and/or closeted. My experience with couples like this is that the partner who is most "out" reacts with frustration and tension—frustration because he doesn't want to live in denial and hiding anymore and tension because he may fear that his

partner will abandon him for a woman if he is bisexual or simply to be alone.

5. *Age discrepancy.* In some couples, one man may be a decade or two older than his partner. Despite lack of support sometimes by their families and friends, these couples are usually quite complementary: the younger man is attracted to the maturity, financial stability, and protection of his partner, while the older man is attracted to the youthful appearance, promise, and playful nature of his partner. They may not fully appreciate that they are at very different stages of the male life cycle. Strain results if the younger man does not evolve as well as his partner expects toward self-sufficiency and self-fulfillment; if the older man becomes overly controlling and dominating of his partner; if the older man becomes possessive and jealous of his partner's friendships with male peers or if the younger man decides to leave the relationship to be on his own.

6. *Fatherhood.* One or both may have children from a previous relationship, usually but not always noncustodial. Their challenges are much like other stepfamilies in that the biological father and the stepfather may be uncertain of their roles and responsibilities toward the child or children. Both the child and the father's partner may be threatened by each other and compete for love and attention of the father/partner. The true nature of their father's relationship with his partner may be a private matter or the child or children may be "out" with their friends.

7. *HIV/AIDS.* In some gay male physician couples, one is or both are living with HIV/AIDS. Relationship symptoms are invariably rooted in loss: of health and physical livelihood, companionship, work (partially or totally), autonomy, privacy, financial independence, sexual intimacy as it once was, self-esteem, and sometimes personal dignity. With newer antiretroviral drugs, especially the protease inhibitors, HIV-positive individuals are not only living longer but also enjoying a remarkable quality of life.

Lesbian Couples. Some of the particular issues faced by couples composed of two women include:

1. *Interdependence and independence.* Some couples must do a lot of negotiating around how much closeness and distance they want with each other. In its most extreme form, couples suffer from fusion or enmeshment and do not have a clear sense of individuality with each other.

2. *Coming-out issues.* This results in conflict if the two women are at different stages of accepting and disclosing their sexual orientation. It is hard to proclaim your couplehood and receive support from family, friends, and colleagues if you are in the closet. One may be quite happy to settle down while the other may cherish her freedom, or may be questioning her commitment to another woman.

3. *Sexual concerns.* There may be a discrepancy between the two women in how often they make love or whether they make love at all. Many lesbian couples are no longer erotic with each other but are very physically affectionate. This may be acceptable to each of them. An unknown number of lesbian women have histories of sexual abuse and sexual assault, usually perpetrated by men, and the emotional consequences of this are serious and far-ranging. Hence, even when they move into a secure and healthy lesbian relationship, they may have trouble trusting others, lack sexual self-esteem, may have arousal and orgasm inhibitions, and feel anxious and phobic. Individual and couples therapy can be very helpful.

4. *Motherhood.* Some lesbian physicians have a child or children by a previous marriage, by a consensual covenant with a male friend, by artificial insemination or other cutting-edge reproductive technology, or by adoption. Some physicians may not have children themselves but have stepchildren with another woman who has children. Their relationship may have suffered enormous strain if there has been a protracted and costly fight with the partner's ex-husband for custody or access. There may be added strain if their geographic community is not very progressive, and the two of them and the children do not receive much endorsement.

5. *Separation concerns.* These are really no different from hetero-sexual separations except that societal support is often less forthcoming, and if the lesbian community is quite small, it is hard to be protective of one's psychological space, to safeguard territoriality, and to meet others. It is not unusual for some lesbian women who were once intimate partners to be friends afterward. When a couple has children, it is important to get good therapy (individual, couple, and family) throughout the separation and good legal counsel.

Helping Couples

There are seven ways that colleagues, friends, and families can be helpful to couples.

1. *Recognition of relationship difficulty and unhappiness.* This is one of the most common challenges for physician couples. When only one of the individuals is concerned, and this is not uncommon, it behooves that individual to let his/her partner know. Possible warning signs include:
   - Inner feeling of tension, unhappiness, irritability, or sadness
   - Vague physical symptoms, eg, headaches, gastrointestinal troubles, backache
   - Increased use of alcohol or other drugs
   - Persistent thoughts of separation
   - Unexplained illness in a child
   - Relationship symptoms, eg, bickering, withdrawal, unresolved arguments, physical violence, avoiding lovemaking, distancing from the partner
   - Outside relationship or affair with someone else

2. *Attempting to make changes on their own.* Trying to listen more attentively and less defensively, getting a babysitter and going out more together, setting aside time to talk each week, drawing up a budget together, and stopping drinking if that's a problem are ways a couple may attempt to make changes on their own. Despite much evolution of sex roles, it is still most often the woman who initiates discussion about the relationship. Most men will engage

in some discussion, but some won't because they can't see a problem, minimize it, or refuse to discuss it. In these marriages, it is only at the point of separation that the man "gets it."

3. ***Barriers to accepting the need for professional help.*** Most men, including physicians, recoil from talking about their intimate relationship with an outsider. Here are common statements from male physicians:

   - I'm a smart man, I'm a doctor, surely we can fix these problems ourselves.
   - Are our problems that bad?
   - My parents went for counseling—great help that was—they split up.
   - What can a counselor do? What do they know? Most of them are pretty screwed up themselves.
   - We can't afford it. And I'm too busy to get away from my practice.
   - I'm not going to air my dirty laundry in public.
   - If we go to counseling, you and the counselor will probably both get on my case about my drinking.
   - You're into this counseling thing—I don't understand all that talk and feeling stuff.
   - Most psychiatrists I know are not real doctors or are kind of weird—and their own relationships are hardly the paragon of success, if they even have a relationship.

And many physicians, women included, feel a sense of failure and stigma if they are having troubles in their relationship. This may have to do with their perfectionistic nature and that they find medicine a rather unforgiving and judgmental profession that does not accept humanness in its practitioners.

4. ***Kinds of help that are available.*** There are a range of professionals who can help physicians who are having relationship problems: psychiatrists, psychologists, social workers, family counselors and therapists, the clergy, and some family physicians. Most employ a conjoint approach, ie, they see both individuals together. They may or may not schedule one or more visits with each individual alone for detailed personal, medical, and family

histories. Their goal is to help the individuals have a better understanding of what is going on, what is causing the conflicts or unhappiness, what may be some of the possible forces from their respective backgrounds that are at work, and what may be some current forces that they have not recognized. They do not take sides but rather aim to facilitate more wholesome communication. Their support and commitment may help to ease misunderstandings and demoralization. If the therapist is a psychiatrist and diagnoses clinical illness in one or both of the individuals, he or she may suggest medication to augment and ease psychotherapy. The outcome of successful therapy is clarity and decisiveness for each partner. If the relationship is viable, both individuals will feel much better together. If the relationship is no longer viable, both individuals should be able to separate with less pain and more dignity, and the therapist can assist with that process.

Conclusion

Most physicians would like an intimate relationship with someone. The responsibilities of medical work—long working days, interruptions in the evening or weekends, sick patients, uncertainty of reimbursement for one's services, and the altruistic nature of physicians—can put much strain on the everyday workings of a relationship. Many physicians in intimate relationships feel torn and guilty and want more balance in their lives, including the sustenance that comes with a healthy relationship. All physicians must strive to give only so much to their work so that they have time, energy, creativity, and some capacity for humor for their partners and family. All physicians who are experiencing unrelenting or intermittent yet recurring strain in their relationships should fight their feelings of shame and seek professional help. Even caretakers need care from time to time!

Suggested Readings

Beck A. *Love Is Never Enough: How Couples Can Overcome Misunderstandings, Resolve Conflicts, and Solve Relationship Problems Through Cognitive Therapy.* New York: Harper & Row; 1988.

Charles SC, Kennedy E. *Defendant: A Psychiatrist on Trial for Medical Malpractice.* New York: Free Press; 1985.

Gabbard GO, Menninger RW. *Medical Marriages.* Washington, DC: American Psychiatric Press; 1988.

Myers MF. *Doctors' Marriages: A Look at the Problems and Their Solutions.* 2nd Edition. New York: Plenum; 1994.

Myers MF. *How's Your Marriage? A Book for Men and Women.* Washington, DC: American Psychiatric Press;1998.

Sager CJ. *Marriage Contracts and Couple Therapy.* New York: Brunner/Mazel; 1976.

Scarf M. *Intimate Partners: Patterns in Love and Marriage.* New York: Random House; 1987.

Sotile WM, Sotile MO. *The Medical Marriage: A Couples Survival Guide.* New York: Carol Publishing; 1995.

Tannen D. *You Just Don't Understand: Women and Men in Conversation.* New York: William Morrow; 1990.

Chapter 6

Depression and Anxiety

Mamta Gautam, MD, FRCP(C)

Mood and anxiety disorders are the two most common types of psychiatric conditions experienced by physicians. In addition, physicians can develop adjustment disorders with depressed and/or anxious mood. This chapter will focus predominantly on mood disorders. Anxiety will be discussed as a feeling state that may be part of a mood disorder. In addition, some of the same psychological factors that promote depression may also contribute to anxiety.

Background

Depression occurs commonly in the general population. Being a physician does not provide any specific immunity against depression. In fact, it may likely make one more vulnerable to depression. Recent data suggest that up to 17% of the population will develop a depressive episode at some point in their lives. The prevalence of depression in physicians is not clearly defined. There are several studies in the literature. However, some of them address psychiatric illness overall and not just depression; some are outdated, having been carried out in the 1960s and 1970s; others lack appropriate control groups, have a small sample size, or have inherent bias. In general, these suggest that physicians have rates of depressive disorders at or somewhat above the general population rates; trainees are especially at risk. It is especially important to be aware that, among women physicians, the lifetime risk of some depressive and anxiety disorders is substantially higher, just as it is for women in the general population.

Depression in physicians may often go unreported. Physicians do not admit to these problems and often do not seek help. Others ask their psychiatric colleagues for informal advice in the "hallway consultation" and so go unrecorded. Many other physicians self-treat. In one study of psychiatric problems in women physicians, 20% of the depressed women physicians disclosed that they had self-prescribed antidepressant medication. I recently reviewed the 100 most recent outpatient charts in my clinical practice and found that 78% of the physician patients had already started themselves on an antidepressant medication before being seen by me, on their own initiative, without the advice or knowledge of their family physician. As one said, *"I've watched many of my own patients struggle with depression, and then improve so dramatically with medication. It looked so easy, so seductive. I wanted to feel better, too. The SSRIs are great—effective, few side effects... and just sitting there in the sample cupboard, waiting for me."*

There is a serious risk of suicide if depression is not treated. One in seven patients with recurrent severe depression commit suicide. Fifty to sixty percent of those who complete suicide suffered from a mood disorder. The high suicide rate among physician patients is alarming. Studies suggest that the rate of suicide in physicians is 1.5 times greater than the rate for the general population for males and three times greater than the general population for females. Chapter 7 provides more information about suicide in physicians.

Depression and Anxiety

Depression and anxiety commonly present together in clinical practice. From 60% to 90% of depressed patients have one or more associated symptoms of anxiety, such as worrying, somatic or psychic anxiety, phobias, or obsessive-compulsive features. Anxiety symptoms can be severe and disabling. One patient described her feeling state: *"My hands shake as the nurse asks me to see the next patient. I feel almost paralyzed. I don't think I will be of any help. What if I don't know what to do for the patient? What if I miss something? What if I go blank? I read the presenting complaint over and over again and can't seem to get up to go to the patient. I can't stop ruminating about missing something big. I just want to lie down and not have to get up."*

There is considerable overlap between anxiety and depressive symptoms. Anxiety can also show up as agitation, insomnia, weight loss, or somatic complaints. Mood and anxiety disorders may share some pathophysiology, since many therapies are effective for both. With our growing recognition that depression complicates all anxiety disorders, and that anxiety complicates all depression, selective serotonin reuptake inhibitors (SSRIs) are becoming the standard first-line treatment for such patients. The symptoms resolve progressively with continued therapy. Anxiety is resolved earliest, often in the first week, followed by improvement of intellectual impairment and somatic complaints. Improvement of depressed mood, fears, and insomnia may not occur until the third or fourth week of treatment.

The presentation of coexisting anxiety and depressive symptoms usually suggests greater severity of illness and chronicity, and a poorer response to therapies. Some of the same risk factors are seen for both mood and anxiety disorders (family history, certain personality traits, etc).

Risk Factors

The risk factors that predispose physicians to depression are many and varied. Risk factors for major depression in the general population include:

- Gender – major depression is twice as likely in women
- Age – peak age at onset is 20 to 40 years
- Family history – the risk is 1.5 to three times higher with positive family history

- Marital status – separated and divorced people have higher rates; married males have lower rates than unmarried males; married females have higher rates than unmarried females
- Negative life events – these often play a role, especially in earlier episodes of recurrent depressive illness

Biological Risk Factors

Biological factors that make physicians more vulnerable to mood disturbances include the following.

- *Lack of sleep* – This is the number 1 complaint among physicians. They work long hours on end and have frequent nights on call. They average two to four hours of sleep during a night of call; experts agree that we need at least eight to 10 hours of sleep each night. This limits their ability to cope in situations with high demands and high levels of stress.

- *Poor eating habits* – Too often, the physician is unable to eat regular, well-balanced meals. Meals are skipped or quickly put together. Fast foods from hospital cafeterias, coffee shops, or vending machines are consumed. During long, busy nights on call, extra meals or caffeine are used to help stay awake.

- *Poor level of fitness* – Busy physicians have little time for fitness for themselves. There is always something or someone more urgent, and they promise to take time for themselves later. Later, they are exhausted and cannot get started once they stop, or anticipate another long day ahead, and decide to rest instead.

- *Positive family history of psychiatric illness* – Some physicians are genetically predisposed to psychiatric illness. A positive family history of mental illness is strongly correlated with psychiatric illness in the physician.

- *Physical illness* – Depression is very common in physicians with physical illnesses, either severe, sudden, or chronic illnesses. Physicians who are no longer able to maintain the previously high level of functioning after the illness, such as with a stroke or heart attack, are especially at risk.

Psychological Risk Factors

Physicians tend to share common personality traits, which lead to similar issues and struggles (see Chapter 4). The following traits are the ones most frequently associated with depression in physicians.

- *Need for perfection* – Some physicians want to be perfect and do all that they can. They are conscientious, attend to all possible details, and do their utmost to meet their responsibilities. Thus, they cannot delegate and find it hard to slow down, relax, or do less than what they see as the right thing to do.

  Case Vignette. An internist asks for help because he has a lot of difficulty supervising interns and residents at his clinic. After they have seen a patient, and completed an exhaustive history and physical examination, they review the case with him. He has to return to the patient and redo the entire assessment, because he needs to reassure himself that nothing has been missed. His clinics are very lengthy, the nurses and residents complain, and his family is upset because he never gets home before his children are in bed at night.

- *Marked sense of responsibility* – Physicians tend to be very responsible people, take their duties seriously, and often feel a sense of responsibility for things that are not under their control. They try to solve problems and feel guilty when they cannot fix everything.

  Case Vignette. A family physician completes a very busy day. Later in the evening, she calls all the patients whom she has seen that day, to make sure they have completed the blood tests she ordered and filled prescriptions she wrote for them, or ask if they have any questions about a medical procedure they have booked for the next day.

- *Need for control* – Physicians generally like to be in control, of themselves and of their environment. They become anxious if they feel out of control, and struggle to stay in control. They try to take control in all situations, even if it is not necessary or appropriate. Sometimes, this is open and aggressive. Yet, it is equally controlling if done in a passive manner, sacrificing their needs for others, unconsciously attempting to control that others approve of them.

- *Need for approval and discomfort with approval received* – Physicians typically need to please people and want to be liked. In trying to please everyone, they may end up feeling that they have really pleased no one. When they get approval or praise, they dismiss or minimize it because they feel uncomfortable with it.

- *Chronic self-doubts* – Some physicians doubt themselves and at times lack self-confidence. These physicians fear that they are "just faking it" and that, any day, their cover will be blown, that people will realize just how little they know. They feel that they have been lucky so far, and managed to get away with it, but could be easily found out.

- *Ability to delay gratification indefinitely* – Physicians are often experts in delaying gratification. They put off earning real salaries like their friends from college to go to medical school. They kept promising to do something once they got into medical school, then once the exams were over, then once they finished call, then once they got into the residency, and so on. Eventually they feel that they worked so hard and deserve things and want the best immediately. They can then overextend themselves financially and feel further stressed.

  > **Case Vignette.** One young physician worked hard to set up his practice and was proud of its success. Shortly after he moved his family into a big house, he decided to buy the lakeside cottage of his dreams. He became increasingly frustrated and resentful when he had to work so hard to keep up with the payments that he could not take time off work to go to the cottage and enjoy it.

It is important to realize that these traits are not inherently a problem. In fact, they are generally major factors in the success of the physician, serving a very adaptive role. Yet they can easily become risk factors for depression or anxiety, if too extreme or if used too rigidly. Unconscious and experiential factors are felt to contribute to the high rates of depression within the medical profession. Some authors have proposed that, for a subset of doctors, choosing to study medicine is a response to a need to compensate for emotional neglect or parental impotence in childhood. This may have resulted in lower self-esteem and contributed to emotional distress and illness.

Social Risk Factors

Physicians are subject to a number of special demands.

- *Patients* – Each physician deals with a small but definite group of patients who can be demanding, dissatisfied, and unappreciative, and dealing with this group is emotionally draining.

- *Scrutiny* – Many people, from colleagues and other health care workers to licensing boards and governmental agencies, are looking over the physician's shoulder and judging his/her performance.

- *Occupational hazards* – There is a serious risk of contracting illness and disease, such as AIDS, hepatitis, or tuberculosis; of being victimized by workplace violence or by sexual harassment; or of managing despite sleep deprivation.

- *The business of medicine* – Physicians are rarely taught business skills in their training, so it is common for them to feel stress in carrying out the business activities of a practice.

- *Maintenance of competence* – Physicians need to keep up with new information and knowledge by attending meetings and managing a large number of journals and books.

- *Organizational changes in health care* – Recent changes in the health care system have led to reductions and redistribution of funds, hospital closures and restructuring, forced retirement, loss of geographic flexibility, and loss of autonomy and independence.

- *Issues specific to women* – Women physicians have minority status and thus face discrimination and scapegoating; not being invited to or being ignored at meetings; not being listened to or taken seriously; being depreciated for their family commitments; having their academic contributions devalued or dismissed; and having few mentors and role models.

Diagnosis and Clinical features

Major affective disorders are characterized by one or more episodes of major illness involving a prominent and persistent disturbance of mood. Once a diagnosis of depression has been made, it is important to differentiate between unipolar major depression and bipolar (manic-depressive) disease. Unipolar disease is 10 times more common than bipolar illness. In bipolar illness, the patient is prone to hypomanic or manic episodes in addition to depression. This is an important distinction, since these patients are at risk for developing a manic episode in response to their treatment for an episode of depression. This will require concomitant treatment with mood stabilizers.

In a manic episode, the essential feature is an elevated or irritable mood, with symptoms such as hyperactivity, excessive activity with little use of judgment, pressured speech, inflated self-esteem, flight of ideas, distractibility, and decreased need for sleep. The manic patient with the obvious symptoms of psychosis or dysfunction is easily diagnosed. The patient with hypomania may be more difficult to identify. One must always ask about such symptoms in a patient presenting for the first time with depression. A positive family history is very helpful, as bipolar illness has one of the strongest familial patterns of any psychiatric illness.

The essential feature of a depressed episode is a depressive mood or pervasive loss of interest or pleasure, associated with symptoms of sleep and appetite disturbance, change in weight, psychomotor agitation or retardation, decreased energy, feelings of guilt and worthlessness, and thoughts of suicide.

Among physicians, there are five early danger signs of so-called burnout, which may be a precursor to a depressive episode. These are:

- An increase in physical problems and illnesses
- More problems with relationships
- An increase in negative thoughts and feelings

- A significant increase in unhealthy habits, such as overeating, not exercising, smoking, increased alcohol intake, or lateness at work
- Fatigue or exhaustion

Treatment

Barriers to Accessing Care

Physicians generally use intellectual defenses to protect themselves from painful emotions. These defenses can be a major cause of delay in seeking help. Physicians often seek help only during a personal or professional crisis, such as the death of a patient, a malpractice suit, family breakup, or acknowledgment of an addiction. Below are some of the defenses that can serve as a barrier to receiving care.

1. *Denial* – Physicians deny that any problem exists. ("There is nothing wrong with me. Patients get sick, not me.")

2. *Minimization* – Physicians convince themselves that the problem is much smaller or less distressing than it really is. ("OK, I have a problem, but it can't be that bad. I still manage well at work.")

3. *Rationalization* – Physicians find an excuse or a reason to explain away the problem. ("OK, I do have a problem, but it's only because I haven't had a vacation for a couple of years. Once I get a break, I'll be fine.")

4. *Reaction formation* – Physicians try to give their patients and other people around them all the attention and care they would have liked to receive.

5. *Displacement and sublimation* – Sometimes, physicians work harder when they feel dissatisfied with their life or feel overwhelmed by demands. They resort to what has always helped them to feel better about themselves, their work, and what also helps to distract them from the upsetting issues. This works because they just do more of something they like, feel more productive, and achieve more, and because it is socially acceptable and even admired to work harder.

Treatment Options

Significant advances have been made in the understanding of depression and approaches to treatment. For mild to moderate, nonbipolar, nonpsychotic major depression (far and away the most common variety seen), pharmacotherapy and several specific forms of psychotherapy have proved to be equally effective. There is no *a priori* reason to select a particular treatment course for physician patients; rather, it is preferable to allow the patient his/her choice of specific treatment option after the advantages and disadvantages of each are explained carefully. Since major depression is often a recurrent illness, a history of a good response to a previous treatment (in the patient or even a family member) might steer treatment selection toward that particular treatment.

There are several distinct classes of antidepressant medication, all with good efficacy and many with fairly minimal side effects. Physicians may be particularly desirous of avoiding certain side effects (eg, cognitive impairment or tremor), and this may determine initial drug choice. A patient who has not responded to a particular drug may still improve on another drug from a different class or even from the same class. Light therapy (phototherapy) may be a somatic yet nondrug option for physicians with a seasonal pattern to their depressions, especially if there are particular concerns about medication side effects or privacy (ie, pharmacists or others knowing about prescriptions).

Interpersonal and behavioral-cognitive psychotherapy are two specific forms of psychotherapy that are generally time-limited, practical, and focused on current difficulties, aspects that may make them especially appealing to some physicians. Some physicians express a fear of or distaste for engaging in open-ended psychotherapy or of having their early lives explored. If an intimate relationship is a major stressor for the depression, or it is sinking under the weight of a depression, couples therapy may be warranted. In general, the beneficial effects of medication are seen somewhat earlier than those of psychotherapy, although psychotherapy is eventually as effective and carries a far lower side effect burden. There is some controversy in the field about whether psychotherapy affords any protection against future depressive episodes; medication certainly does not appear to. Many experts in mood disorders recommend a combined approach to treatment incorporating *both* pharmacotherapy and psychotherapy.

Sixty to seventy percent of patients with depression will respond to initial treatment with monodrug therapy (usually after four to eight weeks of treatment) or to a completed course of psychotherapy (usually 12 to 20 sessions or about 12 weeks). Of the 30% who do not respond to initial treatment, the majority will improve on an alternative approach, and upward of 90% will eventually recover fully. Thus, the prognosis of major depression is among the best of any medical illness of similar severity.

Special Considerations in Treating the Physician Patient

Treating a physician patient can present certain challenges. Physicians are different in some ways from other patients, yet they are not so different in many others. This is a unique therapeutic situation, in which the patient is often as well trained as the treating physician, and it can be intimidating because he/she does not present himself/herself as the usual lay patient. It is hard for physicians to be patients. Many physicians deny problems and have difficulty initiating treatment. This leads to delayed seeking of treatment, and the problem is then often more serious. The insecurities of physicians may make them fear judgment, fear exposure, and feel a sense of guilt and personal failure. In their struggle for control, physicians may try to direct their own treatment. Some physicians self-diagnose, self-medicate, and self-refer. They can be reluctant to follow advice. Some of them refuse to accept that they are ill or to adopt the sick role, and studies show that 10% to 25% of physician patients leave hospital prematurely. They also discontinue medications prematurely and are less compliant with follow-up treatment.

The treating physician can have several reactions to having a physician as a patient. This may provoke insecurities for the treating physician, who may feel inferior and incompetent and doubt his/her abilities. The patient is seen as special and can get poorer care, such as fewer family interviews or a shorter hospital stay. The patient may be mistakenly assumed to know more than he/she does about psychiatric care, and so inadequate information is given. Sometimes the opposite reaction ensues, with the treating physician feeling superior and wanting to compete with the patient. In other situations, there is a strong identification with the patient; the problem hits close to home, and the therapist may feel threatened and deny or avoid the problem, or minimize the illness. Sometimes the treating physician likes the patient and inappropriately wants to be his or her friend.

Below are some specific suggestions for dealing with the physician patient.

- Respond quickly to requests for help. Most physicians have already waited too long before they ask for help.

- Encourage and help them to obtain a family physician. They may need a complete medical evaluation, and they often have too few supports and resources.

- Ensure confidentiality. Reassure the patient of this to help settle fears. Clarify what is required under mandatory reporting; all else is confidential.

- Be empathetic, and acknowledge their courage and strength in seeking help.

- Discuss who is in control – treatment should be a collaborative effort. Take charge, make decisions, and ask direct questions when appropriate, but don't undercut patient autonomy and self-esteem by doing so. At the same time, allow the patient to be "just a patient" and not feel like he/she has to be his/her own doctor too.

- Treat like any other intelligent patient. Special treatment is usually poorer treatment.

- Anticipate the patient's defense mechanisms, and do not allow them.

- If hospitalization is required, ensure that the patient stays in the hospital for the complete treatment course, monitor closely to ensure medication is being taken as prescribed, and follow up after discharge.

- Identify and understand your own reaction to the patient. Be confident and set and maintain appropriate boundaries.

- Avoid sharing of more personal information than you would with other patients (in other words, generally not too much).

- Recognize that what you hear will have an impact on you, and learn to expect and deal with this. Learn to disengage from their pain.

- Care for yourself – take vacations, use social supports, consult with colleagues. Be a good role model for your physician patient.

Prevention

Since physicians are very reluctant to seek help for themselves, it is crucial for colleagues to recognize the signs and symptoms of depression. A conscious change in the culture of medicine is crucial, to foster an environment in which stress is recognized as normal and is openly addressed, and help is offered without judgment.

From the start, this needs to be addressed in medical school. A careful selection process will help to choose well-rounded, emotionally healthy individuals who are better suited to the demands of medicine. Students can be taught about the stresses inherent in medicine, depression, substance abuse, and the problems of overworking. They can be taught self-awareness, the need to care for themselves, to seek support, and to watch out for each other. The importance of a balanced life outside of medicine can be emphasized. In particular, students need to know of the increased vulnerability of women in medicine to depression. These messages need to be continued regularly throughout training and afterward through continuing medical education. Practicing physicians always benefit from the reminder to lead balanced lives.

Physicians must be encouraged to watch out for their colleagues. They can look for warning signs and learn to be comfortable in reaching out to help. It is especially important to be vigilant of colleagues who are vulnerable because of history of depression, who have had life stresses such as marital problems or onset of physical illness, or who are more erratic or withdrawn at work. Physicians need to learn to be more comfortable in reaching out to a colleague about whom they have concerns and assisting him/her to seek help. Covering up for a colleague does not help that colleague.

Depression, even in physicians, is a very treatable illness. Physicians do well when treated, provided that they are persuaded to complete the course of treatment and are supported in follow-up.

Suggested Reading

Prevalence

Clayton PJ, Marten S, Davis MA, et al. Mood disorder in women professionals. *J Affect Disord.* 1980;2:37-46.

Hsu K, Marshall J. Prevalence of depression and distress in a large sample of Canadian residents, interns, and fellows. *Am J Psychiatry.* 1987;144: 1561-1566.

Pitts FN Jr, Winokur G, Steward MA. Psychiatric syndromes, anxiety symptoms and response to stress in medical students. *Am J Psychiatry.* 1961;118:333-340.

Pond DA. Doctors mental health and mental disturbance in doctors. *N Z Med J.* 1969;69:131-135.

Raskins M. Psychiatric crises of medical students and the implications for subsequent adjustment. *J Med Educ.* 1972;47:210.

Welner A, Marten S, Wochnick E, et al. Psychiatric disorders among professional women. *Arch Gen Psychiatry.* 1979;36:169-173.

Special Considerations for the Physician Patient

Gold N. The doctor, his illness and the patient. *Aust N Z J Psychiatry.* 1972;6:209.

Jones RE. A study of 100 physician psychiatric inpatients. *Am J Psychiatry.* 1977;134:1119.

Remick RA. Refractory depressive illness in physicians. *B C Med J.* 1998;40:153-155.

Waring EM. Psychiatric illness in physicians: a review. *Comp Psychiatry.* 1974;15:519-530.

Prevention

Shortt SED. Psychiatric illness in physicians. *Can Med Assoc J.* 1979;121:283-288.

Wise TN. Depression and fatigue in the primary care physician. *Primary Care.* 1991;18:451-464.

Chapter 7

Physicians and Suicide

Morton M. Silverman, MD

T he question of whether physicians are at increased risk for suicide and whether, in fact, they commit suicide at an increased rate compared to the general population has been publicly debated, the subject of medical journal editorials, and internationally researched for the last 90 years. One of the driving forces behind the interest in this topic is the apparent paradox that physicians, who are trained to respect, promote, and preserve life, would choose to end their own lives prematurely. Medical researchers, epidemiologists, sociologists, and psychiatrists have all tried to explain this phenomenon by citing such contributing factors as personality traits, work habits, predilection for psychiatric disorders, high incidence of alcohol and other drug abuse, subspecialty preferences, and role strain.

Six key research questions have predominated since the earliest published report of high rates of physician suicides in 1903[1]:

1. What is the true physician suicide rate?

2. Is the physician suicide rate different from (ie, higher or lower than) that of comparably matched general populations?

3. Is the suicide rate higher for certain subspecialties within medicine?

4. How does the physician suicide rate compare to those in other professional occupations (ie, lawyers, dentists, veterinarians, pharmacists, etc)?

5. Are medical students and house staff trainees at increased risk of suicide because of stress and role strain?

6. Are there identifiable predictors in medical students or house officers for suicidal behavior in later life?

In the last 25 years, additional questions have emerged: (1) Are female physicians at increased risk for suicide as compared to women in the general population? (2) Are women physicians more vulnerable to suicide because of preexisting or predisposing conditions (which predate medical practice) or because of precipitating conditions (as a direct consequence of being a physician)?

Those concerned with the health and mental health of physicians have asked, "Is there something inherent in the experience of doctoring that impacts the suicide rate? Or is there differential selection, whereby those predisposed to the precursors of suicide (eg, depression, alcohol and other drug abuse, unstable social supports) are attracted to medical school, the pursuit of patient care, and even possibly certain subspecialties?"

Although there is century-old literature on the factors (psychological, biological, sociocultural, and environmental) that might contribute to physician suicides, public and professional attention has mainly focused on the rates themselves.

This chapter will focus on physician suicides in the United States, although reference will be made to studies from other countries that may shed light on understanding the cause and prevention of this behavior. The chapter will: (1) analyze methodology problems in surveillance and epidemiology associated with prior efforts; (2) summarize the existing American literature on physician suicides; (3) offer conclusions about prevention based on risk data; and (4) suggest research efforts to inform future discussions of this topic.

Surveillance and Epidemiology

Inquiries by epidemiologists, suicidologists, clinicians, and professional organizations almost always begin with concerns about "how many," "when in the life cycle," and "by what means." I will argue that major inconsistencies in surveillance, definitions of inclusion groups (medical students vs house staff vs practitioners vs retirees), definitions of age group for inclusion and comparison, collection methodologies, and statistical analytic techniques have hampered and hindered definitive statements and conclusions.

Before we can hope to identify those physicians at increased risk for suicide (and, indeed, they do exist) in order to provide preventive therapeutic interventions, we must first answer the basic questions of "how many," "when," and "by what means." Developing profiles of at-risk physicians and clarifying predictive risk factors based on analyses of those who have died by suicide are the first building blocks toward developing intervention protocols.

Methodologic Issues

In the last 30 years, many researchers have raised concerns about the need for sound methodology in the study of physician suicides in order to answer the basic research questions highlighted above.[2-7]

My review of the existing reports on physician suicide rates highlights at least four major epidemiologic survey methodologies that have not received consistent attention in the existing literature: case finding, case definition, sampling bias, and the need for statistical rigor in carefully comparing physician rates to matched national rates (see Table 7-1 on page 98). These concerns exist in the foreground, whereas the problem of studying a low-base-rate phenomenon such as suicide remains in the background.

Few existing studies can be compared because their findings derive from widely varying study approaches and techniques. For example, the identification of physician suicides has been based in separate reports on the review of coroner's death records, newspaper obituaries, state medical society newsletters, family reports, hospital records, anecdotal reports, and medical school alumni newsletters. Obviously, there remains great room for error in accurately reporting not only the true number of suicides that occur and are labeled as such, but

Table 7-1
Methodologic Problems with Physician Suicide Studies

1. Unstandardized and haphazard case finding techniques
2. Inconsistent case definitions
3. Unmatched comparison groups (age, race, and gender)
4. Nonrandomized study time intervals (sampling bias)
5. Poor recordkeeping
6. Unrepresentative samples and cases
7. No investigation of accidental, unintentional, and undetermined causes of death
8. Scarcity of standardized epidemiologic and statistical tools and techniques

Adapted and modified from Silverman.[51]

also those that are "masked suicides" and labeled as something less stigmatizing.

Case Finding. Although accidents (including motor vehicle crashes) still account for more deaths than suicide does in the United States, there is some question as to whether many accidental deaths, or even homicides, are mislabeled, disguised, or masked suicides.[8-13] Few, if any, studies in the literature have attempted to account for the incidence and prevalence of accidents as a "proxy" measure for physician self-destructive behavior. Single-driver motor vehicle crashes, single-pilot aircraft crashes, hunting shootings, and single-driver boating crashes occur at regular intervals among physicians, but these causes of death are often excluded from discussions of physician suicides. Whether they should be is open to question.

Most researchers agree that the standard for certification of death should be the county coroner's or medical examiner's report, although this document may not always provide accurate information about the true cause of death.[11,14] Many published studies of physician suicides do not utilize either of these data sources.

Most investigators have relied on American Medical Association (AMA) obituary records for their source of data. The AMA learns of physicians' deaths through national newspaper clipping services: suicides that are not reported in the local papers would not be included in AMA records. Furthermore, information concerning cause of death is usually obtained from family members or associates and, because of the expense involved, seldom from death certificates. *JAMA* will not publish the cause of death in a suicide case if the family requests it, unless it has already been published elsewhere. In a number of published articles on this subject, the AMA editor in charge of maintaining these death records has been quoted as saying that the *JAMA* obituaries are not valid statistical data, because they tend to underreport the true incidence of suicide in physicians, even more than do statistics based on death certificates.[6,15]

Hence, it is safe to say that there is underreporting of physician suicides in those studies that depend on AMA death data, despite efforts by two research teams that actually rechecked missing and questionable entries from the available AMA datasets they used. Their rechecking increased the accuracy to 95.0% of all physician deaths.[16,17]

Case Definition. There has been a lack of rigor in defining who is a "physician." Standards for case definition have varied widely, including the inclusion of medical students and house staff in the definition of practicing physician. Other studies have included retirees in the physician suicide pool, which then alters what one might be able to identify as professional risk factors for the development of suicidal behaviors. Other studies have arbitrarily used a cutoff age of 64 years for inclusion in the study.

Statistical Issues. The concept of 95% confidence intervals (95% CIs) for analysis of low-base-rate phenomena with low numbers of index cases is essential in analyzing the reliability and validity of the existing reports in the literature. With only approximately 100 physician suicides per year, it is very difficult to extrapolate rates with any degree of confidence. There is a fair degree of uncertainty when dealing with small numbers, especially regarding the small annual number of female physician suicides and the small number of suicides per subspecialty area. The 95% CIs identify the margin of error and allow for ranges when dealing with small numbers.

The use of the 95% CI underscores the concern that if we are to be certain that the physician rate exceeds the population rate, the suicide incidence of the general population must fall outside of the 95% CI of the physician suicide rate.[18] Unfortunately, no study I found in the literature uses 95% CI limits to compare physician suicide rates to general population rates. The standard mortality ratio (SMR) expresses the ratio of the rate of suicide in the physician sample to the rate of suicide in the matched comparison group for the same time frame. The SMRs can then be compared across studies. Unfortunately, only a very few studies provide significant data to accurately determine this ratio. I have tried to calculate SMRs for as many

Table 7-2
United States Physician Suicide Rates

Authors	Period	Scope	No. of Suicides (Gender)	Physician Crude Rates per 100,000 (Gender)	General Population Crude Rates per 100,000 (Gender)	Method of Detection	SMR*
Editorial (1903)[1]	1891-1903	US	519 (M)	39.7 (M)	NA	Unspecified	NA
Knopf (1923)[54]	1912-1921	US	398 (M)	27.0 (M)	NA	AMA records	NA
Emerson and Hughes (1926)[55]	1925	US	61 (M)	45.4 (M)	NA	AMA records	NA
Dublin and Spiegelman (1947)[56]	1938-1942	US	326 (M)	38.7 (M)	37.6[†]	AMA records	103
Public Health Service (1963)[57]***	1950	US	48 (M)	28.7 (M)[‡]	24.1[‡]	Death cert.	119
Dickinson and Martin (1956)[58]	1949-1951	US	191 (M)	31.1 (M)	30.3	AMA records	103
Powell (1958)[59]	1937-1956	Tulsa County, OK	5 (M)	83 (M)	27	Newspapers	307
Blachly et al (1963)[60]	1950-1961	Oregon	8 (M)	30.3 (M)	32.4	Death cert.	94
Craig and Pitts (1968)[7]	1965-1967	US	211 (M)	38.3 (M)	34.1 (M)[†]	AMA records	112
			17 (F)	40.5 (F)	11.4 (F)	AMA records	355
			228 (M/F)	38.4 (M/F)	34.1[†]	AMA records	113
Blachly et al (1968)[15]	1965-1967	US	249	33	38.4	AMA records	86
DeSole et al (1969)[33]	1965-1968	US	291	33	38.4	AMA records	86
Thomas (1969)[61]	1948-1969	Johns Hopkins	14	49.9	NA	Alumni records	NA
Rose and Rosow (1973)[6]	1959-1961	California	48 (M)	77 (M)	38 (M)[§]	Death cert.	203
			1 (F)	18 (F)	16 (F)	Death cert.	113
Pitts et al (1979)[17]	1967-1972	US	49 (F)	40.7 (F)	11.4 (F)	AMA records	357
Steppacher and Mausner (1974)[21]	1965-1970	US	489 (M)	30.9 (M)	26.9 (M)	AMA records	115
			41 (F)	33.6 (F)	10.5 (F)	AMA records	265
Rich and Pitts (1980)[62]	1967-1972	US	544 (M)	35.7 (M)	34.6 (M)[§]	AMA records	103
De Hart (1974)[20]	1966-1971	US	645 (M)	32.9 (M)	32.9 (M)	Maine	100
Bruce et al (1968)[38]	1947-1966	US	35 (M)	NA	NA	Anesth. society	150

Modified and expanded from Rose and Rosow, 1973.[6]
NA = not available.
* Standard mortality rate (observed rate/expected rate x 100).

[†] White men, aged 25 years and over, United States.
[‡] White men, aged 20 to 64 years only.
*** Excludes >65 y/o.
[§] Aged 15 to 64 years.

studies as possible (Table 7-2), although my review of these studies revealed that few met the criteria for a reliable means of data gathering and valid statistical analyses.

Probably the most significant problem with the reporting of physician suicide rates during the past century has been that of failing to used matched age, race, and gender populations. For the first half of the 20th century, the largest majority of physicians practicing and dying in the United States were white men. Although this probably remains the norm even today, the number of female and ethnic minority physicians has increased dramatically in the last 40 years. Hence, it is no longer epidemiologically correct to assume that all the physician deaths in the AMA death files are white men over the age of 25 years (as was assumed in a number of the earlier studies). If one wants to accurately calculate the physician suicide rate in the United States, the AMA physician suicide cases must be first classified by gender (male vs female), age (into 10-year age spans as uniformly reported by the National Center for Health Statistics and World Health Organization), and race (white vs African-American vs other). Only by segregating the suicide deaths into this grid can the physician suicide rates be accurately compared to matched national suicide rates by age, gender, and race. I am aware of only one study that reports the ethnic breakdown of its sample[19] and of two studies that identify suicides in five-year age groupings.[20,21]

Such an analysis would allow for a distinction between physician suicides that occur during years of medical school vs training vs practice vs retirement. Such an analysis would then begin to address issues of the contributions that role strain, personal stressors, environmental risk factors, onset of psychiatric illness, and social and professional stressors might play in the etiology of suicidal behavior in physicians. Needless to say, such an elegant analysis of physician rates by comparison to matched national samples according to age, gender, and race may not be possible because of small numbers in some cells of the grid. Nevertheless, such a careful analysis would be able to definitely answer comparative questions about physician suicide rates. It is only through such a detailed analysis that we can begin to identify risk conditions and risk factors that place physicians at increased risk for suicidal behaviors. Without such an analysis, we will not be able to answer persistent and plaguing questions about whether certain subspecialties do, in fact, have higher suicide rates than other subspecialties.

Suicide Rates

Suicide is, fortunately, a rare event, accounting for only 1.4% of all deaths in the United States in 1996 (the last year that official National Center for Health Statistics data were available at the time this chapter was written). There are approximately 31,000 suicides per year in the United States. Hence, accurate assessment of death determination is essential for calculating precise suicide rates, because of such small numbers. In order to gather sufficient numbers to arrive at statistically significant findings, it is often necessary to conduct multiyear studies. Such studies can often blur occasional annual increases or decreases in the overall suicide rates for a certain population.

There were 249 recorded physician suicides in 1965 to 1967[15] (two years); 530 (489 male, 41 female) between 1965 and 1970[21]; 49 female physician suicides in 1967 to 1972[17] (five years); and 554 male physician suicides in 1967 to 1972.[16] Relatively speaking, physician suicides account for approximately 2.72% to 3.03% of all the male physician deaths in the United States annually[7,17] and 6.52% of all the female physician deaths.[16] Hence, there are approximately 100 physician suicides per year, or, as often stated, the equivalent of an average medical school class per year. This number per year is statistically relatively small and difficult to analyze once you begin to categorize these deaths by age, gender, race, location, and specialty. In summary, case finding, case identification, and case reporting are essential surveillance techniques to help ensure accurate calculations of rates.

The more recent studies (albeit 30 years old) indicate that male physicians overall do not have a greater risk for suicide compared to white males over the age of 25 years,[7] but that the female physician suicide rate in the United States (and in Europe) appears to be three to four times higher than the white female suicide rate over the age of 25 years.[7,17,22-25]

As Table 7-3 indicates, the mean age at suicide for male physicians is in the late 40s, whereas the general male population shows higher rates among those 65 years of age and older. For women, the mean age also is in the 40s, albeit a few years earlier than for the male counterpart. These ages do not correspond with the general population suicide profiles. Of note is that the mean age appeared to increase from the reports of 1968 to 1979. Unfortunately, I am not aware of any more recent data to confirm a trend.

Table 7-3
Mean Age of Death by Suicide

Gender	Mean Age	Study
Male	48.8 ± 0.96	Craig and Pitts (1968)[7]
	51.3 ± 0.60	Rich and Pitts (1979)[16]
Female	41.8 ± 3.07	Craig and Pitts (1968)[7]
	47.8 ± 2.0	Pitts et al (1979)[17]
All	48.8	Blachly et al, 1968[15]
	49.3	AMA/APA (1987)[63]

The more recent studies have reported male physician rates as being similar to matched national rates for white men older than 25 years. However, female physician rates have been found to be four times greater than matched national rates for white women over the age of 25 years. The female physician suicide rates have actually approached the male physician suicide rates. Hence, in the 20th century, during the last 95 years, the focus on physician suicides has shifted from why physicians kill themselves at increased rates, to why women physicians have an extraordinarily high suicide rate compared to matched samples of females in the general population.

Inasmuch as suicide rates are linked to age, the use of "median" ages in comparing "pooled" physician suicide rates to sex-matched national data of the white population aged 25 years and older is statistically imprecise. Furthermore, the assumption in these analyses was that all the reported deaths occurred in white physicians. The collapsing of all the deaths into a number that was compared to a derived rate for white men and women older than 25 years does not allow for the identification of demographic subsets of physicians who might be most at risk for completing suicides.

Female Physician Suicides. If the classic studies by Craig and Pitts[7] and Pitts et al[17] suggest that the female physician suicide rate is comparable to male physician and general male population suicide rates, and is statistically significantly higher than female suicide rates in the general population, then what might place female physicians at higher risk for self-inflicted and self-destructive behaviors? Some studies[26] found that the suicide rate for single female physicians was broadly similar to that of other professional women (lawyers, scientists, writers, nurses, pharmacists, physiotherapists). Of note is a study by Silverman et al[27] that found the suicide rate among graduate female students to be higher than that of matched controls, and the higher rate continued to increase with age. This raises the possibility of a broader phenomenon that affects the population of academically gifted and career-oriented women in the United States.

Research in the last 25 years[26,28-31] indicates that female physicians may share the same vulnerabilities to psychiatric illness and expression of professional problems as do other female professionals (lawyers, scientists, nurses, and pharmacists). Those identified psychiatric illnesses that predominantly affect female physicians are major depressive disorder and substance abuse.

Specialty Studies. There exists a body of literature that suggests that psychiatrists,[2,7,16,23,33-36] otorhinolaryngologists,[7,15,33] anesthesiologists,[7,15,24,33-38] and ophthalmologists[7,15,33] are at increased risk for psychiatric illness and/or suicide as compared to other specialties.

However, the best statistical analyses of the existing United States literature on physician suicides by specialty area do not consistently or reliably demonstrate that any particular specialty is more prone to suicides than another. In short, upon reanalysis of published studies, there does not appear to be any statistically significant differences between the suicide rates among the subspecialties. This conclusion is supported by the fact that these studies suffer from the statistical and epidemiologic shortcomings outlined above (ie, small sample sizes, case finding, etc). Although generating a great deal of speculation, conjecture, and gossip over the years, the few anecdotal reports in the literature of the late 1960s do not provide enough data to allow any meaningful statistical analyses.[7,15,35,38] It is fair to conclude that it is not the specialty per se that contributes to a physician's risk status, but rather what preexisting and predisposing risk factors that physician possesses that are brought with the physician into the specialty.

Medical Trainees. In preparing to write this chapter, I found a multitude of references to medical student stress, residency level stress and strains, and role pressures of physicians. Physicians have been written about, talked about, investigated, probed, and psychologically analyzed for close to 50 years in systematic peer-reviewed studies and medical journal editorials.[39,40] Studies of physician suicides, physicians as patients, physicians as psychiatric patients (inpatient and outpatient), physician stress and role strain, and the increased incidence and prevalence of alcohol and drug abuse, depression, and anxiety have been published.[41] Because of small sample sizes and low numbers of deaths, it is fair to say that the suicide rate among medical students and residents in training is not higher than that of age-, race-, and gender-matched controls in the general population.[7,42] See Chapter 10 for a discussion of particular stresses on medical trainees.

Why Do Physicians Commit Suicide?

Physicians and Role Strain

As DeSole et al[33] noted in 1969, "most explanations for the higher rate of suicide among physicians are either inferential or speculative, based on the available statistical data, and are not based on actual case studies of individual instances of physician-suicides." Such reports are just beginning to appear,[43] but there is no consensus regarding the format and methodology of these psychological autopsy studies. DeSole et al championed the concept of role strain as contributing to the suicide rate in physicians. Role strain exists when there are gaps "between expectations and performances, between promise and delivery, between 'values and norms'... Role strain is intensified if the person is highly committed to his role and the role requires that he function at a maximum level of competence at all times."[33]

Role strain then involves at least three areas of challenge for the physician to master:

1. Inordinate time and work demands
2. Huge sense of responsibility for human life and death
3. Inadequate and inconsistent psychological supports[34]

It is apparent that the blame as well as the resolution for these challenges lies with the individual, the profession, society, and the social support network. From the perspective of the individual, one has to wonder which comes first: substance abuse and/or psychiatric illness (often in the form of depression) that leads to vulnerability to role strain, or role strain leading to alcohol or other drug abuse possibly coupled with a depressive disorder. From the perspective of the medical profession, there seems to be a clear indication to improve upon our teaching, training, and monitoring of the socialization process into the practice of medicine, the type and consistency of messages we provide the public about our invincibility as well as vulnerabilities, and our healthy development of, and respect for, a balanced life. As will be discussed later, the profession has an obligation to its members to provide education about signs and symptoms of suicidal risk.

Physicians and Psychiatric Disorders

Suicide is highly associated with psychiatric illness. In fact, close to 90% of all suicides have diagnosable major depressive disorder and/or substance abuse (alcohol or other drug abuse).[44-46] Existing literature suggests that those physicians who are prone to psychiatric illness are also at risk for suicide. This finding is not significantly different from the existing literature regarding the general population. Hence, most researchers conclude that "psychiatric illness is as necessary a condition for physician suicide as it is for anyone else."[41]

Once again, the limitations of these studies of psychiatrically ill and suicidal physicians are that they are not systematic, randomized, or consecutive. Nevertheless, despite many reports in the literature attempting to delineate relative rates of psychiatric disturbance and vulnerability among physician subgroups, it probably is reasonable to conclude that the risk of suicide in physicians is highest for those physicians with a family history of psychiatric illness or a preexisting psychiatric illness prior to their entrance into medical practice (Table 7-4). In addition, Sakinofsky[26] speculates that the knowledge of toxicology coupled with ready access to lethal drugs increases the potential for impulsive suicidal behaviors that can be often fatal.

Table 7-4
Psychiatric Disorders Associated with Physician Suicide

- Major depressive disorder
- Bipolar affective disorder
- Alcohol and other drug abuse
- Anxiety disorders, including panic disorder
- Borderline personality disorder

Based on references 15, 17, 28, 29, 63, 64, and 65.

Risk Factors and Prevention

The AMA and the American Psychiatric Association conducted a case-control study in 1980 to 1981 using the psychological autopsy method where the background, personality and psychosocial circumstances of the deceased were described. The data were obtained from five states by interviewing the next-of-kin, friends, and colleagues.[47,48] Arizona, California, Michigan, Oregon, and Pennsylvania, comprising approximately 24% of the US physician population, were selected for the study. Of the 1,258 deaths during this two-year period, they identified 24 suicides, 128 possible suicides, and the remaining 1,106 deaths from other causes. Selected for personal interviews with family members were 223 deaths. They included all of the suicides and possible suicides, as well as a random sample of 71 of the deaths from other causes that were posted in 1980 and the first half of 1981.

Interviews were successfully completed on 61, or 27% of the deaths selected for follow-up. Most of the unsuccessful attempts were the result of inability to locate next-of-kin or other survivors, rather than reluctance of widows or others to be interviewed. Although it is easy to criticize the findings based on a small sample size, this study did provide some counterbalancing findings to those previously published, suggesting that a more rigorous project to study this problem is indicated. Retrospective analysis based on interviews of relatives and associates of 15 of the physicians who took their own lives reveals no unexpected difference between the life courses of these physicians and those of 36 physicians who were perceived to have died of natural causes ("naturals"). There were unexpected similarities, however.

No substantial difference, for example, was found in use of alcohol or other drugs between the suicides and the naturals. Thus, 27% of the suicides and 36% of the naturals drank daily, and only 13% of the suicides and 19% of the naturals ever drank more than they did at the time of their death.

Another area where suicides did not differ from naturals was in their tendency to overwork. Half of all the deceased physicians, regardless of the cause of their death, were deemed to be "workaholics" by their spouses and others who were interviewed.

The suicides did manifest special vulnerabilities and were seen to have experienced events and circumstances that were not characteristic of physicians who died of natural causes. Eighty-six percent of the suicides, for example, had sustained personal and professional losses in the immediate past, but none of the naturals had.

With respect to financial matters, 60% of the suicides and only 22% of the naturals were said to have been financially worried. There were even greater differences in attitude toward their own medical careers: 20% of the suicides and 52% of the naturals were "deeply satisfied" with their careers, and 13% and 30%, respectively, were "content," but 33% of the suicides, and none of the naturals, were said to have been "bitterly dissatisfied."

Respondents were asked whether they believed the suicide deaths were foreseeable or preventable. In 53% of the cases, they were "definitely" foreseeable and in 33% of the cases "possibly" foreseeable. But, while 60% were viewed as "possibly" preventable, only 7% — one case — was apparently "highly" preventable. If the physician had been in psychiatric treatment, foreseeability was substantially increased, especially if there was hospitalization for depressive illness. Of principal suicide clues, mood was cited most often—in half of the cases.

Interviewers commented that psychiatric treatment alone, or at an earlier time of life, does not seem to necessarily protect against suicide. If anything, the information indicated that therapists, colleagues, and family need to be much more vigilant about this danger, and more aware of the importance of support systems while the physician is in treatment. It appeared that, too often, friends and family members seemed to believe that because "he's seeing a psychiatrist, we don't have to be concerned or bothered with him any longer."

Yet, there were too few cases of suicide investigated to develop a valid profile of the suicidal physician. A more complete picture would require interviewing additional cases of physician suicide, together with in-depth analysis and correlation of both existing and new data. They concluded that "the information at hand is suggestive at best. It does indicate, in summary, that being depressed, having financial problems, experiencing major personal or professional losses, being dissatisfied with professional life, having a less than responsible attitude toward patients, being uncooperative with colleagues, and deriving little satisfaction from family relationships, can be signals of impending suicide. A physician who sends out more than one of these signals may well be a candidate for prompt collegial concern and meaningful offers of help and support."[49]

Consequences of Suicide

All suicides are tragic in multiple ways, and suicide by physicians may leave an especially devastating wake. In addition to the effects on the surviving loved ones and friends, physicians who kill themselves also directly or indirectly harm their patients by abandoning them and leaving them with many unresolved feelings.[50] Physician colleagues and other health professionals who worked with the physician who completed suicide often experience feelings of anger and guilt for not having prevented the outcome. Suicides among trainees may be especially devastating because of the survivors' lack of previous exposure to suicide and the close bonds (and identifications) often formed among fellow students or residents while in training.

Future Research Directions

The limitations in the extant studies described above highlight the need for more rigorous and clinically valuable studies in the future. The following are my recommendations for what future research studies should do.

1. Rigorously define the sample by level of training, age, gender and racial distribution, and other demographic variables (geography, marital status, etc).

2. Rigorously determine cause of death in all cases where the death certificate may be ambiguous—single-driver motor vehicle accident, unnatural death, drowning, asphyxiation, boating accident, accidental gunshot wound, and unintentional overdose.

3. Determine physician suicide rates by subsamples based minimally on age, gender, and race. Method of death would be an additional category. Ideally, it would be interesting to also parse out subspecialty categories and regional distribution.

4. Calculate standard mortality ratios in order to develop a common reporting language across all studies.

5. Include 95% confidence intervals for the reporting and comparison of suicide rates.

6. Conduct national studies over longer time frames (minimally five years; ideally 10 years) in order to reduce the large statistical uncertainty associated with estimating physician suicide rates from small-sample data (ie, individual states or regions).

7. Conduct prospective studies of female medical students to better understand the factors that might be contributing to their increased suicide rate.

8. Study suicide attempts in physicians because of their high morbidity and statistical association with future suicidal behaviors.

As I have discussed elsewhere: "it is essential that future studies go beyond the first epidemiological steps of 'counting heads' and address the more intriguing questions of what other variables are associated with or may contribute to suicidal behaviors ... and how can they be modified or prevented."[51]

Yet, major obstacles to the initiation of new studies remain. They include the following:

- the inherent frustration and difficulty in studying low-base-rate phenomena over long periods of time

- receiving sufficient financial and administrative support to continue a project that does not generate new data on a regular basis

- mounting a multiyear project using standardized data collection and data analytic techniques

- receiving ongoing cooperation from various components (ie, state departments of vital statistics, local medical societies, family and colleagues)

- overcoming stigma associated with the accurate reporting and investigation of suicides in physicians

- ensuring confidentiality, dignity, and respect for family, friends, and other survivors of physician suicides

- maintaining access to records and other materials that otherwise would not be coordinated and gathered centrally, including medical records and police records

- "foreseeing the future," such that the survey instruments used are not only adequate to the immediate needs of the project but sufficiently visionary to capture the data that might only become relevant years hence, as we evolve our understanding of the dynamics that contribute to these tragedies.[51]

Conclusion

Most studies to date have been concerned with establishing the rate of physician suicide and comparing that rate to the rate in the general population. Only a very small number of studies have addressed the characteristics of those physicians who do commit suicide. Of note is the Johns Hopkins longitudinal study of medical students[52] and the longitudinal study of undergraduate men at Harvard conducted by Vaillant el al.[53] At present, it is probably fair to say that we still lack an accurate and reliable profile of physicians who are at high risk for suicide, and lack a predictive model to identify physicians at a point where preventive interventions might be applied. Table 7-5 summarizes a composite risk profile based on our current understanding of physician vulnerabilities to suicide.

Table 7-5
Profile of a Physician at High Risk for Suicide

Gender	Male or female
Age	45+ years old (female); 50+ years old (male)
Race	White
Marital status	Divorced, separated, single or currently with marital disruption
Habits	Alcohol or other drug abuse "Workaholic" Excessive risk taker (especially high-stakes gambler; thrill seeker)
Medical status	Psychiatric symptoms (especially depression; anxiety) Physical symptoms (chronic pain; chronic debilitating illness)
Professional	Change in status – threat to status, autonomy, security, financial stability, recent losses, increased work demands
Access to means	Access to lethal medications Access to firearms

Based on data from references 6, 16, 17, 19, 43, and 50.

Implications for the content of continuing medical education courses, board certification examinations, and licensing examinations seem evident. Such content would include the early recognition, diagnosis, and treatment of alcohol and other drug abuse, depressive disorders, and other psychiatric disorders highly associated with suicide and other life-threatening behaviors. Medical societies and subspecialty associations need to better educate their members about the potential dangers associated with risk factors for suicidal behaviors. State and local medical society quality assurance committees and ethics boards need to provide better surveillance and increased access to remedial services. More active impaired physician committees can aid in identifying physicians in need of treatment or monitoring.

The possibility of a significantly higher than expected suicide rate for female physicians (compared to matched controls) must be acknowledged and addressed beginning at the medical school level. We must recognize the importance of providing more female physician role models in medical school and residency training programs. We must figure out how to encourage and support women pursuing careers in medicine. This means lowering roadblocks and obstacles to their achieving satisfaction and equality in their careers.

I would argue that to prevent physician suicides from occurring in the 40s, you need to begin interventions in the 20s, if not earlier. At the medical school level, more needs to be done to ensure early detection, diagnosis, and treatment of psychiatric problems and poor adaptation to new roles and responsibilities. Learning to deal with uncertainty, failure, frustration, unrealistic demands and expectations, and competition begins before medical school but surely increases during medical school, into residency and fellowship training, and well into one's practice years. Learning to cope, trust one's judgment, and make balanced choices and decisions are critical skills to acquire and practice throughout a career.

References

1. Suicides of physicians and the reasons (editorial). *JAMA.* 1903;41: 263-264.

2. Bergman J. The suicide rate among psychiatrists revisited. *Suicide life Threat Behav.* 1979;9:219-226.

3. Carlson GA, Miller DC. Suicide, affective disorder, and women physicians. *Am J Psychiatry.* 1981;138:1330-1335.

4. vonBrauchitsch H. The physician's suicide revisited. *J Nerv Ment Dis* 1976;162:40-5.

5. Goppelt JW. Psychiatrists who kill themselves: uncertainty of sources. *Am J Psychiatry.* 1968;124:1471.

6. Rose DK, Rosow I. Physicians who kill themselves. *Arch Gen Psychiatry.* 1973;29:800-805.

7. Craig AG, Pitts FN Jr. Suicide by physicians. *Dis Nerv Syst.* 1968; 29:763-772.

8. Barraclough BM, Holding T, Foyers P. Influence of coroners' officers and pathologists on suicide verdicts. *Br J Psychiatry.* 1976;128:471-474.

9. Moyer LA, Boyle CA, Pollock DA. Validity of death certificates for certificates for injury-related causes of death. *Am J Epidemiol.* 1989;130:1024-1032.

10. National Research Council (Institute of Medicine). *Injury in America—A Continuing Public Health Problem.* Washington, DC: National Academy Press; 1985.

11. O'Carroll PW. A consideration of the validity and reliability of suicide mortality data. *Suicide Life Threat Behav.* 1989:19:1-16.

12. Rosenberg ML, Davidson LE, Smith JC, et al. Operational criteria for the determination of suicide. *Forensic Sci.* 1988;33:1445-1456.

13. Sainsbury P, Jenkins SJ. The accuracy of officially reported suicide statistics for purposes of epidemiologic research. *Epidemiol Community Health.* 1982;36:43-48.

14. Jobes DA, Berman AL, Josselson AR. Improving the validity and reliability of medical-legal certifications of suicide. *Suicide Life Threaten Behav.* 1987;17:310-325.

15. Blachly PH, Disher W, Roduner G. Suicide by physicians. *Bull Suicide.* December 1968:1-18.

16. Rich CL, Pitts FN Jr. Suicides by male physicians during a five-year period. *Am J Psychiatry.* 1979;136:1089-1090.

17. Pitts FN, Schuller AB, Rich CL, et al. Suicide among US women physicians, 1967-1972. *Am J Psychiatry*. 1979:138:694-696.

18. Carpenter RG. Statistical analysis of suicide and other mortality rates of students. *Br Prev Soc Med*. 1959;13:163-174.

19. Revicki DA, May HJ. Physician suicide in North Carolina. *South Med J*. 1985;78:1205-1207.

20. De Hart C. Suicide by physicians. *J Maine Med Assoc*. 1974;65:32-33.

21. Steppacher RC, Mausner JS. Suicide in male and female physicians. *JAMA*. 1974;228:323-328.

22. Simon W. Suicide among physicians: prevention and postvention. *Crisis*. 1986;7:1-13.

23. Lindeman S, Laara E, Hirvonen J, Lonnqvist J. Suicide mortality among medical doctors in Finland: are females more prone to suicide than their male colleagues? *Psychol Med*. 1997;27:1219-1222.

24. Richings JC, Khara GS, McDowell M. Suicide in young doctors. *Br J Psychiatry*. 1986;149:475-478.

25. Arnetz BB, Horte LG, Hedberg A, et al. Suicide patterns among physicians related to other academics as well as to the general population. *Acta Psychiatr Scand*. 1987;75:139-143.

26. Sakinofsky I. Suicide in doctors and wives of doctors. *Can Fam Phys*. 1980;26:837-844.

27. Silverman MM, Meyer PM, Sloane F, Raffel M, Pratt DM. The Big Ten Student Suicide Study: 10-year study of suicides on midwestern university campuses. *Suicide Life Threat Behav*. 1997;27:285-303.

28. Welner A, Marten S, Wochnick E, et al. Psychiatric disorders among professional women. *Arch Gen Psychiatry*. 1979;36:169-173.

29. Clayton PJ, Marten S, Davis MA, et al. Mood disorder in women professionals. *J Affective Disord*. 1980;2:37-46.

30. Bissell L, Skorina JK. One hundred alcoholic women in medicine: an interview study. *JAMA*. 1987;257:2939-2944.

31. Bissell L, Jones RW. The alcoholic physician: a survey. *Am J Psychiatry*. 1976;133:1142-1146.

32. Willi J. Higher incidence of physical and mental ailments in future psychiatrists as compared with future surgeons and internal medical specialists at military conscription. *Soc Psychiatry*. 1983;18:69-72.

33. DeSole DE, Singer P, Aronson S. Suicide and role strain among physicians. *Int J Soc Psychiatry*. 1969;15:294-301.

34. Ross M. Suicide among physicians: a psychological study. *Dis Nerv Syst.* 1973;34:145-150.

35. Freeman W. Psychiatrists who kill themselves: a study in suicide. *Am J Psychiatry.* 1967;124:846-847.

36. Pond DA. Doctor's mental health. *N Z Med J.* 1969;69:131-135.

37. Ward CF, Ward GC, Saidman LJ. Drug abuse in anesthesia training programs: a survey 1970 through 1980. *JAMA.* 1983;250:922-925.

38. Bruce DL. Causes of death among anesthesiologists: a 20-year survey. *Anesthesiology.* 1968;29:565-569.

39. Mental disturbance in doctors (editorial). *BMJ.* 1969;4:448.

40. Physician heals himself (editorial). *JAMA.* 1971;218:1823.

41. Holmes VF, Rich CL. Suicide among physicians. In: Blumenthal S, Kupfer D, eds. *Suicide Over the Life Cycle: Risk Factors, Assessment, and Treatment of Suicidal Patients.* Washington, DC: American Psychiatric Press, Inc; 1990:599-615.

42. Pepitone-Arreola-Rockwell F, Rockwell D, Core N. Fifty-two medical student suicides. *Am J Psychiatry.* 1981;138:198-201.

43. Lindeman S, Heinanen H, Vaisanen E, Lonnqvist J. Suicide among medical doctors: psychological autopsy data on seven cases. *Arch Suicide Res.* 1998;4:135-141.

44. Dorpat TL, Ripley HS. A study of suicide in the Seattle area. *Compr Psychiatry.* 1960;1:349-359.

45. Rich CL, Young D, Fowler RC. San Diego suicide study, I: young vs old subjects. *Arch Gen Psychiatry.* 1986;43:577-582.

46. Barraclough B, Bunch J, Nelson B, et al. A hundred cases of suicide: clinical aspects. *Br J Psychiatry.* 1974;125:355-373.

47. Sargent DA. Michigan part of pilot study on physician suicides. *Mich Med.* July, 1981:356.

48. Sargent DA. Work in progress: preventing suicide among physicians and other members of the health-care team. *Conn Med.* 1981;45:583-586.

49. AMA Council on Scientific Affairs. Physician mortality and suicide: results and implications of the AMA-APA pilot study. *Conn Med.* 1986;50:37-43.

50. McCue JD. The effects of stress on physicians and their medical practice. *N Engl J Med.* 1982;306:458-463.

51. Silverman MM. Campus student suicide rates: fact or artifact? *Suicide Life Threat Behav.* 1993;23:329-342.

52. Thomas CB. What becomes of medical students: the dark side. *Johns Hopkins Med J.* 1976;138:185-195.

53. Vaillant GE, Sobowale NC, McArthur C. Some psychologic vulnerabilities of physicians. *N Engl J Med.* 1972;287:372-375.

54. Knopf SA. Suicide among American physicians. *N Y Med J.* 1923;117:84-87.

55. Emerson H, Hughes HE. Death rates of male white physicians in the United States, by age and cause. *Am J Public Health.* 1926;16:1088-1093.

56. Dublin LI, Spiegelman M. The longevity and mortality of American physicians, 1938-1942: a preliminary report. *JAMA.* 1947;134:1211-1215.

57. Public Health Service. *Mortality by Occupation and Cause of Death.* Vital Statistics Special Reports, No. 3. Washington, DC: Dept of Health, Education, and Welfare; 1963;53:157.

58. Dickinson FG, Martin LW. Physician mortality, 1949-1951. *JAMA.* 1956;162:1462-1468.

59. Powell EH. Occupation, status and suicide: toward a redefinition of anomie. *Am Soc Rev.* 1958;23:131-139.

60. Blachly PH, Osterud HT, Josslin R. Suicide in professional groups. *N Engl J Med.* 1963;268:1278-1282.

61. Thomas CB. Suicide among us: can we learn to prevent it? *Johns Hopkins Med J.* 1969;125:276-285.

62. Rich CL, Pitts FN Jr. Suicide by psychiatrists: a study of medical specialists among 18,730 consecutive physician deaths during a five-year period, 1967-1972. *J Clin Psychiatry.* 1980;41:261-263.

63. AMA Council on Scientific Affairs. Results and implications of the AMA-APA physician mortality project: stage II. *JAMA.* 1987;257:2949-2953.

64. Murray RM. Psychiatric illness in doctors. *Lancet.* 1974;1:1211-1213.

65. Waring EM. Psychiatric illness in physicians: a review. *Compr Psychiatry.* 1974;15:519-530.

Chapter 8

Substance Use Disorders

Stephen J. Dilts, MD,
Michael H. Gendel, MD

Little is known about the incidence of substance use disorders (SUDs) in physicians, especially about whether physicians differ from the general population in any significant way. The growing body of methodologically sound research knowledge is best typified by the study performed by Hughes et al.[1] They surveyed residents and physicians in practice and found that physicians were similar to the general population in terms of previous experimentation with illicit drugs but were less likely to be current users; alcohol use was higher but may have been similar to that of similar socioeconomic groups. The authors expressed concern about their finding of a high rate of self-treatment with controlled substances. Others also have raised questions about self-prescription starting in residency.[2]

Another example of our increasing knowledge is the work of Frank and her colleagues,[3] who reported the results of a survey of women physicians. They noted that women physicians were less likely to report abstaining from alcohol than were to a matched sample of the general population but also were less likely to binge drink.

Illness Course

The natural course of addictive disorders is often described as chronic, relapsing, and deteriorating over time. Spontaneous recovery occurs at an uncertain rate, usually in response to the addict becoming painfully aware of the damage and cost associated with his or her illness. Multiple-organ-system damage is the rule in late-stage disease, leading to significant morbidity and mortality. The type of substance and route of administration affects the course; for example, crack cocaine dependence develops and progresses more rapidly than alcoholism because of the short half-life and short-lived "high" of cocaine, the quick development of tolerance, and the swift brain perfusion of the smoking route of administration. In contrast, alcohol is more slowly metabolized, its intoxicating effects are more sustained, and its oral absorption is slower and less inefficient when compared to crack cocaine.

The degree to which the course of illness is different among physicians, compared to the general addicted population, is unlikely to be related to biological factors, but rather to the social conditions unique to the profession. Special access to drugs is probably the factor that distinguishes doctors from other sufferers.[1] This is especially dramatic for anesthesiologists, who have access to fentanyl and sufentanyl (two powerful narcotics); few others abuse such drugs, and anyone who does so is likely to have an illness that progresses rapidly because of the unique properties of such medicines.

Another primary social factor that impacts the course of illness in physicians is the degree of scrutiny to which doctors are subjected. This is similar to the situation for pilots and, to some extent, those in other professions of public trust and safety, such as lawyers. The fact that many doctors practice in hospitals gives others the opportunity to observe their clinical and other social behaviors. The potential for early identification, compared to the general addicted population, would appear to be present. This opportunity is often missed because of a variety of factors first noted in the seminal *JAMA* article about "sick physicians," especially the ignorance of colleagues and a conspiracy of silence.[4] Further, work tends to be the last sphere of the doctor's life to be affected by addiction, so that by the time work problems have appeared, the illness may be in its later stages.

However, once the physician is identified as suffering from an SUD and either reported to the state licensing board and/or involved with a physician health program, the course of the illness is markedly altered. Though research on outcomes for physicians is not as methodologically clean as would be optimal, most reports suggest that physicians do better in recovering than the general population.[5] The authors believe that this is primarily because of the implicit or explicit contingency contract between the doctor and the monitoring agency in which loss of license would be a direct consequence of continued active addiction.[6]

Doctors may be the most educated professional group with regard to addiction. There are no data to suggest, however, that this has altered the course of illness either with or without comparison to other professions.

Talbott[7] and others have suggested that, because of the mores and values of doctors, as well as certain personality traits common to them, their illness course may be prolonged or protracted. Among the factors proposed as causing this phenomenon are the difficulty of physicians in accepting the patient role, a need to control treatment rather than come to terms with the vulnerability of being ill, trouble in identifying and expressing emotions, excessive pride or shame, the notion that a physician does not air dirty laundry in public, an intimidating style when challenged, and a strong aversion to asking for help.[7] To this list, the authors add the observation that many doctors, even if in a specialty that may be distant from the field of addiction, quietly believe that unless they concur with a diagnosis and treatment plan, it is likely incorrect. However accurate the above clinical observations may be, the degree to which they actually alter the natural course of addictive disorders is uncertain. These factors are nevertheless relevant because they tend to complicate the process of intervening with and treating addicted doctors.

The prognosis for addictive illness is quite variable. Untreated, prognosis is poor. Reports on the success of treatment in nonphysician populations vary from around 25% to above 60% depending on the population, drug(s) used, type of treatment, and definition of success. The prognosis for physicians who have come to the attention of licensing boards and physician health programs appears to be good, according to all existing reports. No known difference in prognosis exists for those physicians who are not followed up by such agencies vis-à-vis the general addicted population.

Identification/Intervention

Early identification of SUD may prevent both physical and social complications; certainly, consequences can be dramatic if the physician passes out or appears intoxicated at work. The warning signs of trouble can be noticed by family, friends, and colleagues. These are the signs universally shown in adapting to any physical or mental illness, specifically, behavioral withdrawal and mood changes.

Behavioral withdrawal is a common reaction to even the simplest illnesses, such as the common cold. Sick people stop as many normal activities as possible and try to take care of themselves. Physicians are no different and may be noted to stop activities such as socializing in the physician's lounge, attending staff and committee meetings, and accepting social invitations. Their significant others also may report lack of involvement in normal activities, such as attending church and going to events with the children. *Mood changes* also are seen in reaction to illnesses and usually involve depression and/or irritability.

These signs frequently are written off as "just a reaction to stress and being too busy" when, in fact, they are a red flag reflecting a coping system that is not functioning normally and needs attention. These early signs at least should be mentioned to the physician and not ignored. If the signs have progressed to a level of serious concern, some sort of larger intervention is needed. Intervention has become a jargon term indicating a process of gathering concerned parties together to confront the physician after appropriate planning and rehearsing. Frequently, this sort of intervention isn't necessary, and a less confrontational but still successful technique can be used. This involves having one or two concerned people sit down with the physician to outline concerns and to spell out both the consequences that may occur if things don't change and avenues for help such as the state physician health program.[8]

Evaluation/Diagnosis

The overlap and interplay of SUDs with other psychiatric diagnoses as well as with medical conditions is well documented in the literature.[9] The cornerstone of a complete evaluation is the psychiatric interview and associated assessment procedures with a primary emphasis on articulating appropriate differential diagnoses, since the foundation for treatment is an accurate and complete set of diagnoses.

History

The evaluation begins with the medical history, including chief complaint and current symptoms, looking for common indicators of substance abuse: fatigue, sleep difficulties, poorly explained minor illnesses and injuries, behavioral withdrawal from normal activities, loss of work time, and mood changes with depression and/or irritability. The physician must be examined like any other patient, but a degree of empathy and respect for the awkwardness of being a physician-patient is an essential element of creating and maintaining a working alliance.

A detailed substance use history is crucial, including addictive prescription drugs to which physicians have access. Family history may be informative. Collateral information can be extremely helpful if the physician will allow family or colleagues to be contacted. In addition, screening tests such as the questionnaire[10] or the Michigan Alcoholism Screening Test[11] may add further information.

Examination

A thorough mental status examination should be performed to determine diagnoses and assess current level of functioning. For cognitive assessment, a standardized test such as the Mini-Mental Status Exam[12] can be used, but adequate testing of physicians may involve more challenging tasks than those found on such a standard exam, especially if the physician is in a specialty that requires administering mental status examinations on a regular basis.

A standard physical exam is indicated in the process of evaluation or treatment. If the diagnosis is not clear, the exam may reveal stigmata of an SUD, such as needle tracks, infections, injuries, and sequelae of liver disease.

Labs

Initial laboratory studies should include a complete blood cell count and liver function tests looking for markers of alcohol abuse such as elevated mean corpuscular volume or liver enzymes; if possible, a urine drug screen should be collected and tested at a lab that can test for the wide variety of addictive medications to which physicians have access, including fentanyl and its relatives for anesthesiologists. These tests can reveal hidden substance use if the physician is denying any problem but other data suggest it. This combination of history, collateral information, and screening tests provides a biopsychosocial picture of the physician's current status.

Differential Diagnosis

Presentation of the differential diagnosis in a nonconfrontational manner is the best approach to gaining a treatment alliance. If the diagnosis is not clear and the physician denies substance use problems despite other input suggesting such problems, an extended evaluation process may help clarify the diagnosis. This process involves the physician agreeing to be abstinent except for approved prescriptions and permitting random and for-cause urine screens. During this time, a second opinion from another addiction specialist can be helpful both diagnostically and in breaking through denial if present. This extended procedure may last from three to six months.

Contingency Contract

If the diagnosis of an SUD or the need for extended evaluation seems clear and the physician continues to deny it, contingency contracting may be a technique that helps engage the physician. If one or two significant others such as family or office partner/employer agree with the need for engagement, they can participate in a meeting to outline a contract of evaluation, treatment, and/or monitoring, specifying the consequences if the contract is not met. The ultimate threat of a report to the state licensing board is very effective in obtaining cooperation.[6]

Reporting

If the initial exam reveals evidence that the physician is currently impaired and therefore unable to practice or is suicidal/homicidal, then appropriate steps must be taken to ensure the safety of both the physician and of those around, including patients. If the physician is not cooperative and safety cannot be ensured, a report to the licensing board must be considered.

Treatment

The first phase of treatment is evaluation and intervention. Although the process described above sometimes is emotionally difficult for evaluator and physician patient alike, and at times even acrimonious, the importance of the therapeutic tone set during these interactions cannot be overestimated. A warm, accepting, respectful, expert, and no-nonsense approach is key to the therapeutic aspect of these activities. The goal of the evaluation/intervention phase is accurate diagnosis and the securing of appropriate treatment for the physician patient.

The treatment of addictive illness among physicians is typically both intensive and extensive. Most commonly, long-term inpatient and/or residential care is prescribed, especially if the physician is referred by a physician health program, hospital, or licensing board. Little is known about what treatments are recommended for doctors who are not referred by such agencies. In fact, long-term residential care has been so well established as "traditional" in the treatment of addicted doctors that any other form of treatment is controversial. For instance, primary outpatient addiction treatment, whether intensive (several days per week, several hours per day) or not, is viewed with skepticism by some in the field. The Colorado Physician Health Program most commonly refers doctors with addictive disorders to intensive outpatient care at facilities with experience in working with physicians.[13] Comparative outcome studies do not exist at present.

As with other medical illnesses, recommendations for treatment should be based on a clinical assessment of need. Those doctors suffering from alcoholism, central nervous system depressant addiction, or opioid addiction often require detoxification. Most commonly this is an inpatient procedure. The American Society of Addiction Medicine has developed broadly accepted patient placement criteria to guide treatment-setting decisions for detoxification and other aspects of addiction care.

Those addicted physicians who are very resistant to the recommendation for treatment, who have had multiple relapses despite treatment, who are suicidal or homicidal, who are in later stages of addictive illness and/or extreme denial of such illness, who have severe concurrent psychiatric or other medical disorders, or who have no social support are probably best treated as inpatients initially. Indications for initiating treatment as an outpatient are more unsettled. We suggest that factors that augur well for successful outpatient care include continued successful function in most spheres, substantial (and sober) social support, early phases of illness, acceptance of illness, and willingness to do whatever is suggested by authoritative professionals. After the initial phase of intensive care (whether inpatient or outpatient), which typically lasts days to weeks, an extended aftercare program is prescribed, lasting one to two years. Length of treatment tends to correspond with degree of success.

The elements of addiction treatment for doctors are essentially the same as for the general addicted population and are primarily psychosocial. These include confrontation of denial by a variety of means, education about addictive disease, and encouragement to be open and honest with fellow recovering individuals in order to meaningfully profit from their support and advice. Additionally, physician patients often need specific issues addressed, such as their tendency to use intellectual coping strategies. One can use this to advantage by providing information to the physician patient and even assigning him or her to do research on some aspect of addictive illness or treatment. Intellectual defenses may be confronted by techniques geared to evoke emotions. Experiential approaches may be employed to help the doctor let go of the control he or she is used to in the doctor role and to better accept the vulnerable position of being a patient. It is essential to insist that the doctor, while in group therapy, learn to ask for help from peers.

It is often said that addicts listen best to other addicts. Those who work with addicted doctors often say that such doctors listen best to other addicted doctors. This is one argument for specialized treatment, that is, treatment in a program that specializes in working with doctors. Clinicians often find it difficult to treat doctors. The common problems are overidentifying with the physician patient or feeling overly challenged. Overidentification leads to a passive, permissive clinical stance in which the therapist avoids necessary conflict with the patient and is reluctant to cause discomfort. The challenged therapist is unnecessarily demanding, critical, and rigid with the physician patient, sometimes overlooking the doctor's shaky self-esteem and thus risking magnifying self-esteem injury. Whether found in specialized programs or other settings, the clinician seasoned in the care of doctors is an invaluable resource. Clinical supervision is often useful for those treating or monitoring physicians, in order to promote therapeutic neutrality and objectivity.

Family involvement is another cornerstone of addiction treatment for all clinical populations.[14] Compared to most families of addicts, physicians' families may be more prone to humiliation, shame, and feared loss of the addict's livelihood and prestige. They may be in the habit of "enabling" the doctor to avoid the natural consequences of addiction by making excuses or protecting the physician from interactions that would expose the illness. Like others in similar circumstances, a physician's family members often feel deprived and angry. They are likely to be surprised and enraged to find out that, far from returning to the family fold, the newly recovering doctor has a schedule full of outside activities necessary to sustain recovery. By acknowledging feelings, providing support, and educating, family engagement in the treatment process advances the development of a healthy matrix of support for the recovering doctor.

Biological treatments are important adjuncts to addiction treatment for physicians, as for other patients. Disulfiram (Antabuse®) and/or naltrexone (Revia®) for alcoholism and naltrexone for opioid dependence are frequently utilized. More controversial is the use of methadone for opioid addicts, particularly if the physician wishes to continue practicing medicine.

Random urine drug testing is useful with physician patients. Most addiction treatment programs use urine testing for an objective checkpoint in determining that a patient is indeed drug free, and for help in identifying relapse at an early stage. Patients profit from knowing that relapse is likely to be detected. Urine testing for addicted physicians has added benefit if used in contingency contracting. Contingency contracting is a highly effective form of treatment in its own right.[6] The physician who knows his relapse will result in possible licensure consequences is more motivated to abstain from addictive substances.

The concept of monitoring has specific meaning when applied to the recovering doctor. Those addicted doctors whose difficulties are known to hospital credentials committees or licensing boards are usually monitored by those groups in the first years of recovery, most frequently by their requiring random urine testing and asking for reports from those providing primary treatment. Physician health programs, which are experienced in following up the recovering doctor, work with those physicians known to hospitals and licensing boards, but they may also serve many doctors who have sought help confidentially. Physician health programs typically monitor the progress of recovering addicts by urine screening; face-to-face clinical evaluations; obtaining input from family, 12-step sponsor, and colleagues as appropriate; and obtaining reports of those doing primary treatment of the physician. Such clinical monitoring is more sensitive to relapse than urine screening alone and is also more supportive to the doctor in recovery. Many hospitals and licensing boards utilize physician health programs to conduct their monitoring. This arrangement has the added advantage of introducing more distance between the agencies and those actually providing primary treatment to the physician, allowing for more confidentiality.

Psychiatric symptoms, such as depression or anxiety, are almost universal in the actively addicted physician. These symptoms tend to resolve as abstinence is achieved. However, a significant proportion of substance abusers have comorbid psychiatric illness, not simply psychiatric consequences of addiction. Addiction patients with untreated other psychiatric illness have a poorer prognosis than those with SUDs alone.[15] Addicted physicians with substantial psychiatric morbidity should be carefully assessed and followed up. Treatment should be initiated for the diagnosis of any psychiatric illness. Treatment should avoid medicines that have addictive properties.

Twelve-step programs alone are not adequate treatment for SUDs. Most reputable addiction treatment programs nevertheless incorporate the principles of 12-step programs (the fellowships of Alcoholics Anonymous, Narcotics Anonymous, Cocaine Anonymous, and others) in their structure. They do this by teaching such principles, helping the patient apply them to the solution of life problems, providing reading materials, encouraging attendance at 12-step meetings and obtaining a sponsor, and assigning them to work the early steps of the program while in intensive treatment. Physician addicts also find such programs useful, if not absolutely essential to their ongoing recovery and pursuit of "serenity."[16] Some doctors are skeptical about 12-step programs, citing as objectionable apparent religiosity and the endorsement of powerlessness over the drug of abuse. These reasons for rejecting participation in 12-step programs are almost always primarily expressions of fear and shame about suffering from addiction and can be, indeed should be, worked through via the treatment process.

Work-related Issues

If the physician has taken time off work in order to participate in treatment for addictive illness, return to work will be a significant step. For those who suffered impairment in cognitive function as a result of their illness, return to work is predicated on sufficient restoration of that function, such that they are not compromised in their ability to provide safe and competent care to patients. The stability of the physician's condition, in terms of both addiction and any psychiatric or other medical problems, must also be ensured.

Return to work is fraught with danger for newly recovering doctors. For many, it is at work that they will first confront colleagues, powerfully exposing themselves to their own shame and embarrassment and possibly to the actual negativity of others. Many doctors also feel guilty about "abandoning" their colleagues, especially if others had to take over their caseload or on-call demands. Between their assumption that colleagues are angry, and their own sense of responsibility, recovering physicians have a tendency to throw themselves into work. This often threatens the integrity of their recovery program, which is quite time-intensive. Further, exposure to the stress of work adds to the complexity of their vulnerable emotional state. It is important for those treating and monitoring the doctor to anticipate these events. Conferences with colleagues and staff prior to return to work can ease the pain and enhance support during this transition. In such meetings one can provide education about the illness, discuss what can be expected of the returning doctor, and answer questions about how others can help.

Some addicted physicians find recovery to be threatened in association with work, either because of the stress of work or because of specific triggers. Specific triggers may include drugs themselves (as addictive medications are often available to physicians at work) or other environmental cues that may trigger drug craving. Return to work should be preceded by a careful assessment of drug availability in the workplace and planning for how to protect the addicted doctor. If the physician used drugs from the work environment, this is critical. Certain specialists may be even more vulnerable to this problem. Anesthesiologists who use fentanyl or sufentanyl obtain such drugs only at work. A concern has been raised as to whether anesthesiologists with this pattern of drug abuse should ever return to practicing anesthesia; however, in our experience, a carefully structured treatment and monitoring plan allows a successful return to work for these physicians. Nonetheless, in relapses with these substances, there appears to be a high potential for fatalities.[17]

The Americans with Disabilities Act may provide some help for recovering physicians as they approach their workplace. This federal law directs employers, under certain conditions, to accommodate the medical limitations of employees. When the conditions of the law are met, this may allow physician employees to modify their work hours, shifts, or other aspects of work life so that they can participate in treatment and recovery activities without compromising their jobs. Legal consultation is advised for physicians considering whether or not the statute offers protections in their case.

It is essential for recovering physicians to learn to manage work stress and to develop good self-care skills. This is easier said than done. Many doctors have managed work stress by working harder and by delaying or compromising the basic care they need. Counseling may be necessary to help these physicians build self-care and stress management into their lives. It is helpful to ask the doctor to schedule meals, sleep, exercise, time with family, relaxation or meditation, doctor appointments, therapy groups, and 12-step meetings before any work is added to the calendar. These matters should be the girders of a time management plan, onto which work is built. Counseling may also be beneficial in teaching the doctor to appropriately say "no" and to place limits on responsiveness to work demands.

The recovering doctor should seek the advice of other doctors who are further down the road of recovery. Twelve-step programs can be effective in cementing both stress management skills and self-care. The first two steps continually orient the doctor as to the primary importance of recovery activities as compared to other activities, including work. The third helps reduce the stress of any situation that might feel overwhelming. Steps 4 through 9 systematically expand the physician's acceptance of illness and its harmful effects on others, offering maximum opportunity to address shame and guilt. The 12-step fellowships provide robust social support, encouragement, and perspective; all are fundamental needs of the recovering doctor.

Regulatory Issues

Many physicians with addictive illness have come to the attention of their state licensing board, the authority that regulates the practice of medicine. This is a particularly painful position for a physician. Physicians' reactions tend to be dominated by either anger or shame.

When angry, they are furious at the board, feel violated by its investigation, want to discredit the board or its members, and fight with every aspect of the negotiations. When ashamed, physicians want it all to "go away," may fail to respond to the board's process, and are often compliant to the point of failing to make obvious points in mitigation.

To assist the recovering doctor in these matters, it is necessary to understand the reason for the licensing board's involvement. Boards are responsible for protecting the public safety and do so by investigating, when called upon, whether or not a physician has violated a section of the civil law that authorizes and governs his practice. In most states this law is called the Medical Practice Act. If the physician is found to have violated it and to have committed unprofessional conduct, sanctions may be imposed. Sanctions range from admonishment not to conduct oneself again in that manner, to censure, to suspension or revocation of the physician's license. In many states, simply suffering from addiction constitutes unprofessional conduct under the Medical Practice Act. Addicted doctors may commit other unprofessional conduct related to the symptoms of their illness, including neglect of cases or abandonment of patients, violations of professional boundaries, or providing substandard care because of lapses in judgment or cognition. It is necessary to clarify what potential violation the board is investigating. Then it is possible to help the physician confront the problem.

It is helpful to conceptualize the Medical Practice Act violation as one of the consequences of the addiction, further evidence of its unmanageability. These doctors should be encouraged to talk with treaters, monitors, family, and others about their feelings about being involved with the board. Self-defeating attitudes should be confronted. In the United States today, investigation by licensing boards is a common occurrence; it is useful for doctors to regard answering to their licensing board to be but one more aspect of their professional responsibilities. They should obtain legal representation experienced in professional conduct issues for help in responding to and negotiating with the board.

For the addicted physician who has undergone appropriate addiction treatment and has achieved sobriety, the most common outcome of the licensing board process is entering into a probationary agreement with the board. Such an agreement stipulates the violation of the regulatory law and requires the physician to fulfill certain conditions in order to continue to practice. These conditions typically include abstinence from addictive chemicals and participation in recommended treatments. The doctor will be required to have treatment monitoring that will minimally include random urine drug screens and may involve meetings with a monitor or physician health program. Monitoring of the practice may be required, especially in the case in which the board found issues regarding the quality of clinical work. Such agreements usually have a time frame, averaging three to five years, at the end of which the physician may apply for an unrestricted license. Legal representation is advisable for physicians.

It is unclear how, and to what extent, the Americans with Disabilities Act applies to the relationship of a licensed physician to the licensing board. The application of this statute continues to evolve via individual case decisions in various states. Consultation with an attorney experienced in this area of the law is essential for any physician wanting to know if, in his or her case, there are protections offered.

Fitness for Duty and Disability

The question of when a physician is fit to practice medicine is complex. Little substantial scientific study has been brought to bear on this issue. To say that basic cognitive, emotional, and behavioral functions must be sufficiently intact is to beg the question: What degree of intactness is required, for how long should it be present prior to entering or reentering the workplace, and how is such functioning to be evaluated? The question is made more complex by asking about competence to practice, how it can be measured, and how it can be improved.

Rather than take up the task of answering these difficult and sometimes theoretical questions about fitness for duty, we propose a practical guide to approaching the issues as they arise in working with the addicted physician. The degree to which illness, including addiction, affects the ability to work requires clinical assessment. If substantial cognitive, emotional, or behavioral impairment exists, it is best to ask the physician to take time off work until the impact of such impairment can be assessed, even if not undergoing residential treatment that would require leave from work.

In addition to the fundamental clinical evaluation, basic questions can be asked at the time of assessment to orient the evaluator in this area. Does the physician have concerns about their ability to practice; have staff or colleagues expressed informal concern; has any practice group or hospital formally looked at quality of care, and what were the results; has there been any formal action or discipline by any agency regarding the clinical work; have there been recent bad patient outcomes; have there been malpractice claims or suits in the recent past? Although no single response tells the evaluator that the physician is unfit for practice, positive answers alert one to the need for more in-depth evaluation. During the assessment phase, it is also important to talk with spouse and family about their concerns about work impairment. Speaking with colleagues and staff is also essential. If the doctor has a supervisor or clinical administrator, inquiring about work performance is appropriate.

If questions about work performance remain after the above procedures, other steps can be taken. Neurologic evaluation and especially neuropsychological testing can give more information about cognitive function. It is most helpful to consult with a neuropsychologist familiar with the range of performance typical of physicians. However, there is no absolute "physician standard" among these tests. Subtle questions about psychological function or impulse control may be answered by psychological testing, if, for instance, there is a concern about an occult psychosis. Medical and laboratory examination may be required when there are questions about the impact of concurrent medical illness (eg, diabetes, AIDS) or when entertaining suspicions about the presence of another illness (eg, dementing neurologic condition). Further, one may perform a chart review of the doctor's inpatient or outpatient practice. Finally, one can ask that the physician obtain a practice monitor, a colleague who would agree to review either charts or cases with the doctor in order to learn about the quality of work and/or to ensure its quality.

If the physician has been off work in order to enter residential treatment, by the time such treatment is over one usually has a clear idea about his or her abilities and limitations. The above evaluation process should have occurred, and lingering concerns can be approached with the same strategies. As research about physicians' work continues, there is hope for a more specific and standard way to look at work performance.

Generally, a clinical evaluator should not attempt to assess competence because this is better done by those specialized in the field, such as educators. Some states have programs designed to address these issues.

Beyond the clinical question of whether addicted physicians are able to work is the insurance-related subject of whether they are disabled. Whether insured by a private disability carrier or applying for public disability assistance, it is an insurance question because each insurance agency defines what constitutes disability. One must be clear about the policy definition before any opinion about disability can be rendered. With private disability policies, disability may be defined in terms of being unable to perform all the duties of the job or some of the duties. It may be defined as being unable to perform the specific job, eg, neurosurgeon, or a more general job, such as doctor. Whether an addicted physician is disabled will be quite dependent on such definition. Social security disability and worker's compensation delineate specific factors that should be considered when determining disability status; these should be studied as they would apply to a specific case before opining to a recovering doctor whether he or she might meet the conditions of these agencies (social security) or laws (worker's compensation).

When assessing disability, or interacting with an insurance carrier regarding this matter, it is helpful to be clear as to the reason an addicted physician may be disabled. Disability may be caused by active addiction, the need to leave work in order to receive adequate treatment, the need to pursue recovery activities so extensive as to preclude work, the need to recuperate, convalesce or temporarily manage stress, or the need to manage relapse risk. Such reasoning, as it applies to the specific physician, should be articulated in sufficient detail to reveal how his or her condition impacts the conditions governing disability as stated by his or her policy.

Future Directions

Anecdotal information from the various physician health programs uniformly suggests that there is a 90% positive outcome for any diagnosis, although SUDs are discussed most frequently. Scientifically based outcome research is badly needed; to begin addressing this need, the 1996 Physician Health Research Conference was organized. It was the first conference to focus exclusively on research issues and methods for physicians. The conference was initiated by the Department of Psychiatry in the School of Medicine at the University of Colorado Health Sciences Center and the Colorado Physician Health Program. Forty participants represented a wide range of national organizations, and at the end of the conference they agreed to establish a Physician Health Research Planning Group (PHRPG) at the American Medical Association.

The PHRPG has been meeting twice a year and has looked at important questions concerning the lack of uniform standards regarding diagnostic entities, specific treatment and monitoring modalities, and precise outcome measures; in addition, it hopes to address the problem of lack of pooled data. The vast majority of the outcome studies have been from single programs or single states; although these reports may contain useful information, meaningful statistics require the numbers gained by multistate aggregate data.

The PHRPG hopes to promote the creation of a permanent, national interorganizational structure to support research on physician health, illness, and impairment and has started to develop a standardized database that could be the basis for outcome data useful to licensing boards, credentialing organizations, and other groups. The development of the database requires agreement on definitions of slips, relapses, recovery, and other terms.

Suggested Readings

Talbott GD, Gallegos KV, Angres DH. Impairment and recovery in physicians and other health professionals. In Graham AW, Schultz TK, Wilford BB, eds. *Principles of Addiction Medicine*. 2nd ed. Chevy Chase, MD: American Society of Addiction Medicine; 1998:1263-1280.

References

1. Hughes PH, Brandenburg N, Baldwin DC, et al. Prevalence of substance use among US physicians. *JAMA*. 1992;267: 2333-2339.

2. Christie JD, Rosen IM, Bellini LM, et al. Prescription drug use and self-prescription among resident physicians. *JAMA*. 1998;280:1253-1255.

3. Frank E, Brogan DJ, Mokdad AH, Simoes EJ, Kahn HS, Greenberg RS. Health-related behaviors of women physicians vs other women in the United States. *Arch Intern Med*. 1998;158:342-348.

4. American Medical Association Council on Mental Health and Addictions. The sick physician (impairment by psychiatric disorder including alcoholism and drug dependence). *JAMA*. 1973;223:684-687.

5. Blondell RD. Impaired physicians. *Prim Care*. 1993;20:209-219.

6. Crowley TJ. Doctors' drug abuse reduced during contingency-contracting treatment. *Alcohol Drug Res*. 1986;6:299-307.

7. Talbott GD. Denial in chemical dependence: special issues for impaired physicians. *Psychol Med*. 1987;3:349-355.

8. Nace EP. *Achievement and Addiction: A Guide to the Treatment of Professionals*. New York: Brunner/Mazel; 1995:34.

9. Kessler RC, McGonagle KA, Zhao S. Lifetime and 12-month prevalence of DSM-III-R psychiatric disorders in the United States: results from the National Comorbidity Survey. *Arch Gen Psychiatry*. 1994;51:8-19.

10. Ewing JA. Detecting alcoholism: the CAGE questionnaire. *JAMA*. 1984;252:1905-1907.

11. Selzer ML. The Michigan Alcoholism Screening Test (MAST): the quest for a new diagnostic instrument. *Am J Psychiatry*. 1971;127:1653-1658.

12. Folstein MF, Folstein SE, McHugh PR. "Mini-mental state": a practical method for grading the cognitive state of patients for the clinician. *J Psychiatr Res*. 1975;12:189.

13. Dilts SL, Gendel MH, Lepoff RB, Clark CA, Radcliff S. The Colorado Physician Health Program: observations at seven years. *Am J Addict.* 1994;3:337-345.

14. Enders LE, Mercier JM: Treating chemical dependency: the need for including the family. *Int J Addict.* 1993;28:507-519.

15. Mirin SM, Weiss RD. Substance abuse and mental illness. In: Frances RJ, Miller SI, eds. *Clinical Textbook of Addictive Disorders.* New York: Guilford; 1991:271-298.

16. Galanter M, Talbot D, Gallegos K, et al. Combined Alcoholics Anonymous and professional care for addicted physicians. *Am J Psychiatry.* 1990;147:64-68.

17. Menk EJ, Baumgarten RK, Kingsley CP, Culling RD, Middaugh R. Success of reentry into anesthesiology training programs of residents with a history of substance abuse. *JAMA.* 1990;263:3060-3062.

Chapter 9

Disruptive Behaviors, Personality Problems, and Boundary Violations

Michael H. Gendel, MD

Working as a physician has traditionally been among the most gratifying and satisfying of endeavors. Some might argue that changes in the structure of the health care system are diminishing such fulfillment by reducing physician power and remuneration, but, from the time of Hippocrates, finance and power have not been physicians' principal rewards. Fundamental among the activities that lead to gratification are the acts of caring, treating, and, when possible, curing. The technology of the modern age and the pleasure of its mastery, along with improvement in treatment outcomes, have added immensely to the satisfactions of medicine, but the most fundamental satisfactions have never been technical.

Case Vignette. A third-year medical student tearfully reported the death of his patient. A 14-year-old girl had died of interstitial pneumonia, after a long deteriorating course and a final bout of illness in which the student had been a caregiver. In the hubbub surrounding her acute care, the student had noticed that no one took the time to talk with her. He did so regularly. As her illness spiraled downward, she was intubated, never to speak again. Patient and student doctor exchanged notes. He saw the look of fear in her eyes, and the semblance of an appreciative smile on her face when he wrote to her words of explanation or encouragement. One morning she handed him the notebook they used for correspondence, and he found her writing physically disorganized and her thoughts incoherent. Once that day she managed to scribble, "What's going on?" She died that afternoon. When speaking to his attending physician about his experience with his young patient, the student found himself surprised to say that, in addition to being distressed by her loss, he had found caring for her deeply meaningful. More than ever he was sure he wanted to be a doctor.

Connecting with patients, often under powerful emotional circumstances, can give rise to feelings of worth and completion that few other activities can bring. The power to help and the power to be seen as helpful can be intoxicating. Related to such elemental satisfactions, but far from identical to them, are those that come from expressions of thanks on the part of patients and families. At times even society—professional societies, workplaces, communities— can express appreciation for physicians' work. Additionally, there remains some status and prestige in being a doctor. Physicians know that society relies upon them. Further, working as a doctor, like most work, is productive; productive work is inherently satisfying.

Though practicing medicine provides doctors with such a potentially gratifying livelihood, the ethical structure of medicine guides doctors away from their own gratification and toward the benefit of patients. From Hippocrates' "First, do no harm," to the more contemporary focus on avoiding the exploitation of patients, physicians are implored to place their own gratification on the back burner and, furthermore, to guard against a tendency to meet their own needs at the expense of patients. Just as an object's mass alters the gravitational field, medicine's very power to gratify the practitioner may alter the treatment relational field such that the needs of patients become subtly secondary. Under these circumstances, patients become a means to the end of physicians' gratification.

Case Vignette. A 45-year-old male internist treated a younger female journalist for diabetes. She was very pleased with his care and admired his knowledge of her illness and his skill in helping her. When she decided to write professionally about current approaches to diabetes, she asked him if he would consent to be interviewed and utilized as an expert for her article. He was flattered by her attention and respect for him and looked forward to their meetings with a sense that, finally, he was going to receive some public recognition of his expertise. They met several times in his office for this purpose. During some interviews she talked of her own medical problems. The patient noticed that on certain of these occasions it was hard to direct her doctor's attention to her medical complaints, and that he tended to wax on about her illness when in fact she wanted help and advice. She considered confronting him about this, but sensed his need for recognition and that for the present she was a means to that end for him. She liked him and felt sorry that he was evidently so unfulfilled despite his clinical excellence. She dutifully completed her article, but never again trusted him so completely.

Patients mobilize trust in physicians. This trust is essential for their care. It allows patients, even in a first visit, to divulge private concerns, remove their clothes, and allow themselves to be touched. Such trust borders on faith: It is not dependent on the personality of the doctor, past experience with the doctor, or indeed any realistic appreciation of the risk of harm that could come from such a stance. It is a product of the role of the doctor, and of an adaptive suspension by patients of their usual behavioral rules regarding what is appropriate to say and do with a relative stranger. It is an adaptation born of need, the need for help and care. This need for help is the gist of what is often termed the vulnerability of patients. Patients' vulnerability leads—indeed requires—them to cast the doctor in the role of trusted helper. At its essence their trust is unrealistic, not because doctors cannot realistically be trusted, but because the trust has a generalized, all-good, one-dimensional, unvarying quality to which no human being can live up. In the above example, the journalist no longer trusted her doctor in the same way because she had seen the chinks in his doctorly care for her.

Patients' unrealistic feelings of trust toward doctors and doctors' feelings of deep gratification and power with patients can be a potent combination. It can lead both parties to feel special and connected to each other. At its best it is one of life's fine partnerships. Its potential for healing is great. It is also a rich medium in which personality problems of doctors can grow into forms that bring unintended and lasting negative consequences for patients.

Disruptive Behaviors

Personality and Personality Disorders

Both Vaillant et al[1] and Gabbard[2] have published accounts of physician personality traits. Self-doubt, guilt, an exaggerated sense of responsibility, and compulsiveness are common features of doctors' personalities. Beyond these more common traits, it is difficult to generalize about doctors' personalities, much less their personality disorders, though self-doubt and guilt may be fertile ground for, and in certain cases may reflect, Axis II pathology. Despite the stereotypes of the kindly family doctor or the controlling, pompous surgeon, doctors' personalities come in all shapes and sizes.

Usually physicians' personalities are flexible enough to allow doctors to conform to standards of behavior laid down by the profession, be it in the Hippocratic Oath, the Principles of Medical Ethics,[3] the requirements of regulatory law (the Medical Practice Act of each state), or the by-laws of hospitals. Breaches of such expectable behavior may be caused by sufficiently severe personality difficulties, which may include personality disorders (Axis II psychiatric disorders), as well as by a variety of situational, educational, and illness factors. That is, interpersonal functioning may be disturbed by factors other than personality disorders. The presence of a health problem, such as severe physical illness, and including Axis I psychiatric disorders, can also serve to precipitate potential personality difficulties into actual ones. Doctors suffering from active addictive disorders typically appear to have personality disorders, though when in recovery such "disorders" often vanish and always improve.

There is no reason to believe that physicians are less subject to personality disorders than other populations. Personality disorders, by their nature, adversely impact a doctor's ability to consistently know and/or respect the boundaries of appropriate behavior. Exploitative doctors have myriad opportunities to exploit patients. Narcissistically disordered doctors may be liable to have difficulty appreciating the difference between their needs and those of patients, and thus to warp the treatment situation in the direction of their own interests. Borderline physicians may have unstable and volatile relationships with patients. Dependent physicians may be too easily influenced by unhealthy patient demands. Physicians with personality disorders are generally less cognizant of the boundaries of appropriate professional behavior, less able to modulate their behavior, and more vulnerable to the tendency of personality-disordered patients to pull doctors off their professional centers.[4] Even in the best of situations, the interpersonal field of doctors with patients is subject to the powerful force born of gratification and vulnerability. Doctors with personality disorders are sometimes too inflexible and self-centered to effectively and helpfully manage this force.

The gratified doctor-thankful patient is far from the only doctor-patient relationship paradigm. Physicians with personality problems are unusually vulnerable to responding to adversity in maladaptive ways, be the adversity a patient's criticism, a bad patient outcome, a mistake, a threatened professional liability suit, or a crisis in their personal lives. Under such circumstances, these doctors may become inappropriately irritable, unpredictable, withdrawn, or impulsive in clinical situations. They may be more inclined to make poor clinical decisions, or, by virtue of their more problematic behavior, they may provoke their patients to take a less helpful stance regarding their own medical care and self-care. Patients, already vulnerable, will obviously suffer. Their care may be compromised. At the least, the damage to their essential and adaptive trust will be considerable. At worst, poor medical decisions by their erratic doctors or poor decisions by the disrupted patients will have serious adverse medical consequences.

As problematic as personality-disordered physicians are for patients, they can be even more difficult for employers, hospital administrators, office and hospital staff, and regulators. It is the behavior of such physicians that causes problems, though their behavior may clearly reflect certain personality styles and attitudes that are also quite problematic.

Description of Disruptive Behavior

Physicians who exhibit problematic behavior as illustrated by the following case are often termed disruptive physicians:

> **Case Vignette.** Dr Y is a 35-year-old divorced surgeon who came to the attention of his hospital department because of habitually critical and demeaning comments he made to others in the operating room. These comments were usually made to those beneath him in the hierarchy of the OR, but anesthesiologists and fellow surgeons as well could find themselves the target. Because he was an excellent practitioner, few had the wherewithal to confront him, lest he escalate the attack by finding real fault with the work of others and humiliating them. The situation ultimately came to a head when, furious at the actions of a nurse attending the surgery, he threw a hemostat at her that narrowly missed.

The frequency of such severe behavior problems is not well studied. Donaldson[5] found in northern England that 6% of senior medical staff had behavior problems that warranted consideration of disciplinary action. Half of the group left the employer's service; the other half accepted counseling or supervision and remained at work.

Disruptive physicians pose special problems. They create situations in which patients are dissatisfied, staff and colleagues reach their wits' end, and administrators feel paralyzed, caught as they are between the threat of lawsuit by patients and staff and some often unnamed threat elicited by the intimidating doctor. Often such doctors deny to themselves or to others the wrongful nature of their actions. They tend to externalize responsibility for those behaviors they admit, by blaming coworkers, administrators, working conditions, patients, or other events. They resist effective confrontation by setting up covert threats of retaliation or even self-harm. They may overtly use their powerful positions or personalities to silence perceived criticism. They resist the monitoring of their behavior by challenging the authority of those who order it and by finding loopholes in the behavioral requirements. Commonly, they are so sensitive to criticism that any intervention attempt tends to heighten shameful feelings, to which they respond with even more problematic behavior.

Case Vignette *(continued).* After his department chair confronted him, Dr Y accused his administrator of attempting to cover up certain problems in the OR by blaming them on Dr Y. Further, he made note of several bad outcomes from surgeries performed by the chairman. He also painted the complaints of OR staff as transparent attempts to dodge the consequences of their own incompetence. He commented that if the local media knew how poorly the OR was functioning, the hospital would be in for some nasty publicity. His resistance to accepting responsibility for his actions prolonged the negotiations about how to proceed. In the meantime, his operating room behavior deteriorated further. He felt unfairly treated, even ganged-up on, by operating room staff. He dreaded having to work there, but he was too brittle to share his distress, reach out for help or understanding, or admit wrongdoing. Instead he became more gruff and withdrawn but no less critical. His discomfort about who was saying what about him made it very difficult to communicate effectively while operating. Apparently, no patient suffered because of these communication problems, but the possibility of this occurring was on the mind of everyone.

Lawsuits brought by hospital or office employees, malpractice suits brought by patients, and adverse hospital publicity are among the many problems created by the disruptive practitioner. The poor morale of those subjected to the doctor also factors into the cost of failing to address such behavioral problems. When the behavioral idiosyncrasies of doctors begin to affect the ability of other health care personnel to get their jobs done, to affect their rights to work without harassment, or to reduce such physicians' ability to work competently, action should be taken.

Administrators must sort out the truly disruptive doctor from the unpleasant or obnoxious one. According to Horty[6] and Horty and Barker,[7] certain behaviors are considered "actionable" by employers and administrators. These behaviors include personal and unprofessional verbal attacks; impertinent and inappropriate comments written in medical records; sexual harassment of medical/hospital staff or patients; intimidating, belittling, nonconstructive criticism; requiring unnecessarily burdensome activities of staff that have nothing to do with patient care; public criticism of other doctors, hospitals, or personnel that occurs outside of appropriate channels; and refusal to accept medical staff assignments or doing so in a disruptive manner.

Management of Physicians with Disruptive Behavior

Once a physician has been identified against whom action must be taken, two lines of intervention should be considered: administrative management and clinical evaluation. Administrative management must begin immediately. Regardless of the cause of the behavior problem, the goal of ending that behavior is an immediate and long-term need. Individuals in authority must confront such doctors. It is best to do so in a setting comfortable to the administrator. A quiet, matter-of-fact, but firm tone is recommended. The meeting should include a specific account of the problem behaviors, with documentation available. The seriousness of the concern should be emphasized. Clear behavioral expectations, to be implemented immediately, must be articulated. These expectations should also be detailed and specific, regarding both what to do and what to refrain from doing. How the expectations are to be monitored should also be presented. The consequences of failing to agree to the conditions of administration should be made clear, be it suspension or loss of privileges, report to medical licensing board, or others. The doctor should be referred for clinical assessment at this time.

The importance of clinical assessment cannot be overstated. While the management of behavior problems unrelated to major illness or acute stress is heavily reliant on clear behavioral expectations or monitoring, when such problems are mainly caused by illness or stress they will seldom be remedied by behavioral management alone. Evaluation should not be performed by agents or staff of the administrative entity, be it a hospital, employer, practice group, or medical board. To do otherwise would be to invite confidentiality and privacy problems, and to dilute the force of a neutral, independent assessment. Likewise, clinicians who evaluate physicians, under usual circumstances, should not treat them. Accusations of conflict of interest will lessen the force of the treatment recommendations. Many state physician health or peer assistance programs are well suited to undertake such evaluations.

If clinical evaluation reveals the presence of major illness, treatment of the illness is essential. Addiction, mood disorders, anxiety disorders, and general medical disorders demand effective treatment if it is hoped to resolve behavior problems that are downstream from them. Management of acute and overwhelming stresses usually requires professional intervention too.

If evaluation fails to reveal major illness, it may yet yield a picture of personality disorder. It is important to avoid making such a diagnosis until other illness has been ruled out, because, as noted above, other illness may mimic personality disorders and certainly will exaggerate them. Psychological testing is at times useful in making such a diagnosis. Many personality-disordered physicians can be assisted through psychotherapy. It is helpful to refer such doctors to psychotherapists who are adept both at working with personality disorders and at working with physicians. In less skilled hands, such doctors will be much less likely to receive real assistance and will thus be more vulnerable to difficulty managing their behavior.

Case Vignette *(continued).* Dr Y was clinically evaluated and found to be suffering from depression. Additionally, he painfully described a childhood replete with verbal and physical abuse perpetrated by his mother. Dr Y had also recently divorced and was struggling in an unstable relationship with another woman. He was referred for psychiatric treatment. He undertook weekly psychotherapy initially focused on helping him manage the stresses associated with his hospital situation and those stemming from his recent divorce and current relationship. His psychiatrist noted him to be interested in, even hungry for help. He was started on an antidepressant, which quickly ameliorated vegetative symptoms of depression. As he distanced himself from his current girlfriend and negotiated a more civil relationship with his ex-wife, he began to talk about his childhood abuse. At this time, his brittle exterior softened noticeably. Hospital administrators began to hear that operating room personnel found him less difficult and even at times likeable.

Monitoring of behaviorally disordered physicians should continue for a substantial length of time, from months to years, even when improvement is dramatic. Personality and behavior problems do not improve in a linear fashion; relapse of problem behaviors is common. It helps such physicians to know that behavioral guidelines will continue to be enforced.

> **Case Vignette** *(continued).* After several months of looking better, Dr Y again lashed out in the operating room, mercilessly belittling a technician. Now less defensive about himself, he took the technician aside afterward and apologized to him. The incident was reported to his chief, who met with Dr Y and informed him that a single further incident would lead to his suspension. Dr Y accepted this limit and was ultimately able to conform to it.

At times clinical evaluation may reveal a personality disorder that does not appear amenable to treatment, or it may also fail to demonstrate any personality disorder. Some doctors behave badly without fitting into any diagnostic schema, indeed, without suffering from any known disorder. Physicians in these groups are best addressed by administrative management alone, while those with diagnosable or treatable conditions should be approached with treatment and administrative management.

In addition to the package of behavioral expectations and consequences described above as administrative management, organizations can pave the way for better management of disruptive physicians by taking several actions. These include writing bylaws that explicitly address behavioral expectations of doctors, establishing and publicizing a zero-tolerance policy about violations of such bylaws, documenting incidents and trends, educating practitioners about such issues, developing confrontation strategies before they actually need to be implemented, and establishing a track record of confronting physicians whose behavior requires administrative intervention.

Boundaries and Boundary Transgressions

Definitions

As defined by Gabbard and Nadelson,[8] professional boundaries in medicine "are the parameters that describe the limits of a fiduciary relationship in which one person (a patient) entrusts his or her welfare to another (a physician), to whom a fee is paid for the provision of a service. Boundaries imply professional distance and respect, which, of course, includes refraining from sexual involvement with patients." Gutheil and Gabbard[9] describe boundaries as the "edge" of appropriate professional behavior. Boundaries are structures within the physician-patient relationship. In a sense they are theoretical; no one literally trips over them. Boundary theory is a body of work that addresses boundaries and the principles that underlie them. While there is uncertainty and debate about exactly what is and is not appropriate professional behavior, there is no doubt that the distinction exists. Figuratively, physicians at times do trip over, inadvertently or purposely, structures that are essential for permitting the doctor-patient relationship to maintain its helpfulness. It is the potential for the helping relationship to become harmful that brings focus to the boundaries of appropriateness.

Previous sections of this chapter have described conditions that may impact the ability of physicians to maintain the "distance and respect" mentioned here. Powerfully gratifying conditions may prevail that alter the doctor-patient relational field in the direction of doctors' own needs. Personality problems, whether due to personality disorders or to regression in personality function associated with major illness and stress, erode a doctor's capacity to recognize or care about when he or she has violated boundaries of appropriate behavior.

The clearest boundary for physicians involves the issue of sex with patients. The Hippocratic Oath[10] addresses this matter: "I will come for the benefit of the sick, remaining free of all intentional injustice, of all mischief and in particular of sexual relations with both female and male persons." A significant body of evidence exists that physician-patient sex is harmful to patients.[11,12] Direct patient harm is characterized by damage to the trusting physician-patient relationship and a number of common psychiatric consequences such as depression, anxiety, guilt, isolation, and sexual confusion. Physicians may also harm patients with whom they have become romantically or sexually involved by losing objectivity in treating them.

Legal and Ethical Aspects

The vulnerable position of patients, which, as noted in this chapter, begins before the patient and doctor even meet each other, leads to a power differential in their relationship with their physician that reduces their ability to make reasonable decisions about how personally involved they should become with their doctor. Patients are therefore more easily exploited by their doctors, whether intentionally or otherwise. For all these reasons, the American Medical Association (AMA) stated "Sexual contact which occurs concurrent with the physician-patient relationship constitutes sexual misconduct."[13] There is general professional agreement on this issue; it appears to be a clear boundary. Yet, clarity is disturbed as the power of magnification is increased: What constitutes sexual contact? What time period represents concurrence? What determines whether a relationship is physician-patient? What about doctors practicing in rural environments where literally everyone might be a patient? Moreover, who is to answer these questions?

Many specialty medical societies have adopted policies that echo that of the AMA. The American Psychiatric Association, which has called psychiatrist-patient sex unethical since 1973, in 1993 expanded its policy to include former patients.[14] The Medical Council of New Zealand recognized gradations of sexually inappropriate physician-patient behavior in formulating its classes: sexual impropriety involves such things as suggestive comments made to the patient, examination and draping practices that are immodest and intrusive, and making sexually demeaning remarks. Sexual transgression involves inappropriate touching short of sexual relations, such as kissing, or touching breasts or genitals outside of standard examination practice. Sexual violation refers to sexual intercourse, oral sex, anal intercourse, and mutual masturbation.[15]

State legislatures have attempted to answer certain of these questions. In Colorado it is a felony for a mental health professional, including a psychiatrist, to engage in sex with a patient. The Medical Practice Act in Colorado[16] prohibits physician-patient sexual relations, and defines the time period for this prohibition as "during the course of patient care or within six months immediately following the termination of the physician's professional relationship with the patient." It defines sex as "sexual contact, sexual intrusion, or sexual penetration as defined in section 18-3-401 C.R.S." Section 18-3-401 is a section of the Colorado criminal code, that further specifies the definition of those acts. These examples are but one of many states' attempts to solidify the understanding of this, the clearest of the boundaries.

It is clearly important for physicians and patients to be protected by guidelines that are as unambiguous as possible. Attempts to be too specific, however, have their pitfalls, as all legislation and rules run the risk of having unintended consequences,[9] which may unnaturally inhibit physicians in working with patients or may subject them to legal consequences for acts that are not truly unprofessional. This problem becomes even more evident when other boundary issues are considered. Much of the attention to nonsexual boundary problems stems from concern that they ultimately lead to sexual intercourse or other blatant sexual impropriety. This concept is referred to as the "slippery slope" and was derived from examining cases of those who perpetrated sexual misconduct.[17,18] Many physicians who have become sexually involved with their patients previously have engaged in other behaviors that were questionable. These involve not only sexual behavior short of intercourse, but a variety of actions that may reflect disturbance of the usual structure of the doctor-patient relationship. Presumably, as doctors lose their grip on usual professional behavior and bend the rules, they become both less sensitive to appropriate boundaries and more vulnerable to acting out, more dangerously, their own needs with patients. Nonsexual touching, conduct of the physical or psychiatric examination, office practice and appointment hours, fees and collection practices, business dealings with patients, personal relationships with patients, and self-disclosure are all areas of physician conduct that came into focus. Over time, it was recognized that boundary problems of this type could be damaging in their own right, with or without the slide into sexual violation.[19,20] These domains of physician behavior are worthy of the attention given them, but the edge of appropriateness remains difficult to pinpoint.[21]

Conceptual Frameworks

Another component of current boundary theory involves Gutheil and Gabbard's[22] distinction between boundary crossings and boundary violations. Boundary crossings are events in which the usual treatment relationship structure is flexed but without harm to patients. Neither patient exploitation nor physician gratification is involved. These are often events in which failure to cross the boundary would be inappropriate, such as accepting the hand or embrace of an acutely bereaved patient, physically assisting an injured patient, or treating a close friend in an urgent context. Boundary violations, on the other hand, harm or potentially harm patients, and may be exploitative.

The frequency of sexual misconduct is difficult to ascertain, largely because of reliance upon the self-report of physicians, or the reports of patients who complain to state medical boards.[23-25] Both of these methods are likely to underestimate frequency. In 4% to 10% of cases disciplined by medical boards, inappropriate patient contact was the reason. Among doctors who become involved with patients, men greatly outnumber women. Most of these relationships are heterosexual, but same sex contact does occur. Psychiatrists and obstetrician-gynecologists are overrepresented, presumably because of the degree of intimacy that is present in the normal treatment situation.

Several schemas for classifying sexual boundary violations have been offered. Each has its value. The differences often have to do with the patient or treatment sample known to the authors, or the authors' underlying theoretical approach or perspective. Gabbard's psychodynamic scheme uses the categories of psychotic, predatory psychopathy and paraphilias, lovesickness, and masochistic surrender.[26] The psychotic group has lost reality testing and may suffer from delusions about sexual relationships. The group of predatory psychopathy and paraphilias includes those with antisocial or severe narcissistic disorders and those with sexual disorders who involve their patients in their compulsive behavior. They often become involved with numerous patients. Lovesick physicians are those who fall in love with patients, or whose behavior is related to apparently deep affectionate feelings for them. The nature of their psychopathology is often narcissistic or neurotic, and the misconduct is often associated with personal crises. The masochistic surrender group becomes involved in a cycle of being resentfully manipulated by demanding patients into a variety of escalating boundary violations.

Irons[27] uses an archetypal view as means of arriving at a gestalt of offending doctors. He classifies such physicians as a naive prince, wounded warrior, self-serving martyr, false lover, dark king, and wild card. Simon's approach,[17] derived from a forensic perspective, groups such doctors as suffering from personality disorder, sexual disorder, incompetence, addiction or other Axis I mental disorder, or situational reactions. Shoener's schema[28] classifies with a view to the issue of rehabilitation of offending doctors. His categories are manics, sociopaths and those with severe narcissistic personality disorders, those with impulse control disorders, chronically neurotic and isolated doctors, situational offenders, and those who are naive.

The effort to classify is an attempt to bring some coherence to the study of sexual and other boundary violations. The central point is the need to assess each case in order to determine what is wrong, what may be helpful, how dangerous it is for the doctor to continue practicing, and the conditions under which safe practice may be possible.[29]

Case Examples and Discussions

Several case examples illustrate these issues.

Case Vignette. Dr A, was a 45-year-old male pain specialist, was reported to the medical licensing board by a member of his office staff. The staff member came to realize that, with several female patients, Dr A gave prescriptions for pain medicine in exchange for sexual favors. The board had no trouble documenting the allegations. Dr A was evaluated psychiatrically; no Axis I disorder was found, including no substance use disorder. He suffered from antisocial personality disorder. His license was revoked by the medical board.

This case is one of an exploitative, predatory physician who regularly used patients for his sexual gratification by playing upon their vulnerability that stemmed from pain and addiction. There is little debate about how to approach such a physician. Medical boards may examine a case of sexual misconduct with a view to finding mitigating conditions or aggravating factors. Mitigating factors are those facts about a doctor's state of health, mental health, life problems, educational deficits, insight and remorse about his or her behavior, or other circumstances that would cast a softer light on his or her otherwise destructive actions. Aggravating factors are those conditions, such as the knowledge that the behavior was unethical, the personal gain involved, the vulnerable position of the doctor's patients, and the pattern of misconduct, that underscore the purposeful, self-serving, and reprehensible nature of the doctor's actions. In the case of Dr A, there is no mitigation and much aggravation. Any attempt to rehabilitate him, a difficult task, would require a model of treatment that approaches him as a sexual offender. His return to practice would be unlikely.

Case Vignette. A 55-year-old psychiatrist became increasingly preoccupied with a younger female patient whom he had seen for some months. She was going through a divorce, as was he. He found himself becoming increasingly directive with her, offering advice about how to manage a variety of matters; this was uncharacteristic for him, and he realized his patient didn't actually require such concrete help. One day she commented that he did not look well, and he shared with her that he was indeed having a bad day associated with his divorce. She became more dependent on him, and more isolated in her own life. They began to have therapy sessions three times per week, though he typically saw even more seriously ill patients only once a week. At times he met her late, after his usual hours. Her bill mounted, but he did not address this with her. Concerned about her isolation, he offered to accompany her on walks or to movies. She readily accepted. On one of their outings she made it clear that she would accept a sexual overture from him. They had sex on several subsequent meetings. Initially they felt glad to have each other and carried away with the idea of the relationship. Within a few weeks each realized that it was a mistake, and moreover that it made further therapy impossible. They became overwhelmed by guilt. He felt he had harmed her and her treatment; she felt she'd used poor judgment regarding what was best for her and had contributed to the potential professional ruin of her doctor. They terminated both their personal and professional relationships. She was referred to another psychiatrist, and he also entered therapy.

This scenario is one of the most commonly seen. A vulnerable physician and patient follow the slippery slope of less serious or sexual boundary violations to that of a sexual affair. The doctor's interest in the patient is genuine up to a point, and may border on love. He believes his motives to be altruistic, at least at the beginning, and has little insight about the extent of his emotional needs, much less the importance of his addressing them in a healthy manner. He begins to share his problems with his patient, who readily begins to trade roles with him, offering him solace and companionship under the guise of letting him help her. When the sexual relationship is consummated and the romantic relationship seemingly about to flourish, it occurs to both parties (not always so simultaneously) that the whole thing is hollow, a blind alley, disappointing and destructive. Now each is faced with healing a new wound, in addition to the problems each of them faced previously. Of course, the doctor was supposed to be helping his patient with her problems.

Many of these physicians can be helped and are able to return to safe practice. Essential to rehabilitation is for physicians to develop a clear understanding of the power of their position, the vulnerability of their patients, the damage they have caused,[30] and the strength of their own unmet emotional needs. Personal crises must be addressed. Depressive or anxiety disorders should be treated. Monitoring of their practice is usually helpful.

> **Case Vignette.** A recently trained pediatrician had sexual intercourse with the mother of a patient in a back area of a hospital. She propositioned him, and each was overcome, if momentarily, with excitement. He was new to practice, without an active love

relationship, and highly stressed at the time. He appeared naive about the ethics of such behavior, ashamed and sheepish in his approach to evaluation and treatment. Psychopathology was mild to moderate, and responded well to education, psychotherapy, supervision, and clinical monitoring. Followed up for more than a decade, he has had no further problems.

This case presents the more benign area of the spectrum of physician sexual misconduct. Education, clear behavioral guidelines, and help with relatively mild emotional problems are often sufficient interventions.

Case Vignette. A 75-year-old internist, Dr B, began to hug his female patients as they left his office. Two of them complained to his nurse that during the hug they had felt his erect penis pressed against their bodies. Each had known Dr B for many years and were flabbergasted by his behavior, and felt comfortable enough with the office staff to register their complaints. History revealed that Dr B had recently suffered a stroke, though had supposedly recovered completely. Closer examination revealed both some lingering neurologic deficits and a variety of impulse control problems that had arisen since the stroke. He realized there was something amiss in the lack of his usual inhibition. His practice was already very limited in scope, and with assistance he chose to stop seeing female patients. He soon retired.

Case Vignette. A 35-year-old internist, Dr C, was the subject of several complaints to the medical board, which occurred in rapid succession, about his sexual behavior with patients. Several women reported that he rather suddenly had changed his demeanor, talking in suggestive and overtly sexual terms, exposing his penis, and inviting them to have sex with him. At the same time, a female colleague in his department reported to their chairman that he was making unwelcome and rather startling advances toward her. Examination revealed a florid manic state, including a delusion that his semen could cure illness.

Physical and mental illness can directly induce states in which physicians engage in impulsive sexual behavior with patients. The extent to which their problematic sexual behavior can be ameliorated depends on effective treatment of the primary illness.

Additionally, the second case above, Dr C, represents a case of sexual harassment. Sexual harassment is not a primary subject of this chapter but is relevant in discussions of both boundary problems and personality problems. The boundary violated in sexual harassment of a colleague or employee is not related to the structure of treatment, but to the structure of the workplace. Treating coworkers respectfully, allowing them to do their jobs without harassment or a hostile work environment is the responsibility of every worker in that environment and of the organization in which he/she works.

Many of the same factors that predispose to disruptive behavior or boundary violations may also contribute to sexual harassment. Those who engage in sexual harassment require clinical evaluation and administrative management as set forth in the earlier section on personality problems. Additionally, physicians who engage in sexual harassment may be subject to legal action.

It is not unusual for a doctor to be referred for evaluation of another problem, and sexual misconduct is found in the process of assessment.

> **Case Vignette.** A 37-year-old ophthalmologist was seen for problems with depression and suicidal impulses. This condition arose after his most recent arrest for indecent exposure. Many years previously he had been arrested and prosecuted for this act in another state. Close questioning about his behavior as a physician revealed a single instance of having had oral sex with a patient, a woman who offered sex as a means of payment. He was encouraged to report this to the medical board, which he did. His license was revoked. He entered a series of treatments based on a 12-step model of sexual addiction, in addition to individual and group therapy for his paraphilia. He was able to successfully return to practice after years of extensive treatment.

This physician had not involved patients with his paraphilia (exhibitionism), but he had violated sexual boundaries as a symptom of his preoccupation with sexual matters. In some cases, this preoccupation with sexual matters functions like an addictive illness and responds to treatment and group support in a manner similar to the addictions. Treating his depression alone would not have helped the boundary problem, as it too was a symptom, or result, of his poorly controlled sexual impulses.

> **Case Vignette.** A 50-year-old family practitioner had alcoholism that had been progressively affecting his life, but he had never previously been inappropriate with his patients. After a back injury he began to abuse opioids and sedatives. At this point his behavior markedly deteriorated in all spheres—his marriage, relationships with family and colleagues, work habits, and personal hygiene all fell apart. He began to hug and kiss many of his female patients, and proposed an affair with one of them. He later attempted suicide.

Substance use disorders cause deterioration of mood, personality function, behavioral control, and judgment. They often do not affect a doctor's practice until they are in late or end stages. This severely ill physician required extensive treatment in order to attain stable sobriety. Many doctors with this picture are ultimately able to return to practice under careful and aggressive monitoring of their sobriety and office behavior.

The issue of sexual boundary violations is an emotional one. Physician behavior that harms patients is cause for concern and action. Sexual behavior that harms patients also produces alarm and moral outrage in many people. Such reactions are natural and understandable, but they complicate the question of how best to remedy the offensive behavior, protect the public, and help physicians to be in a position to safely help patients. A clearer understanding, based on research, of the effectiveness of treatments for those doctors who violate sexual boundaries should help this difficult situation.

Nonsexual boundary problems can be seen in some of the above examples. Examining the breadth and scope of such problems will not be attempted here. Many boundary problems normally confront physicians.[31] Doctors must learn to examine their physicianly behavior as a part of their practice duties. It is useful for doctors to learn to read their own signs of discomfort, signs that they are operating near the edge of appropriateness. With a good understanding of such internal signals, it is easier to stop and consider actions. Doctors should be encouraged to use empathy, considering how a patient might experience them, as a tool for examining the propriety of their behavior.

Physicians require education about and assistance with the dangers associated with the gratification their work may bring, and help in acquiring the skill to evaluate the question of for whose benefit they are acting, their patients' or their own. Help with assessing and support for managing potentially problematic patient situations can come from supportive and trusted relationships with colleagues and from peer assistance programs. Some situations are also aided by the physician undertaking personal psychotherapy or by arranging supervision of clinical practice by another experienced physician. Physicians who attend to appropriate internal cues and avail themselves of collegial resources are far less likely to have problems with boundary transgressions.

Notes

All case vignettes used in this chapter are based on actual cases but have been heavily disguised to protect the confidentiality of those involved.

I am indebted to Scott McClure, MD, for his assistance in discussing disruptive physicians.

References

1. Vaillant G, Sobowale NC, McArthur C. Some psychological vulnerabilities of physicians. *N Engl J Med.* 1972;287:372-375.

2. Gabbard G. The role of compulsiveness in the normal physician. *JAMA.* 1985;254:2926-2929.

3. Council on Ethical and Judicial Affairs, American Medical Association. *Code of Medical Ethics: Current Opinions With Annotations.* Chicago: American Medical Association; 1996-1997.

4. Gutheil TG. Borderline personality disorder, boundary violations, and patient-therapist sex: medicolegal pitfalls. *Am J Psychiatry.* 1989;146:5970-602.

5. Donaldson LJ. Doctors with problems in an NHS workforce. *BMJ.* 1994;308:1277-1282.

6. Horty J. The disruptive physician. *Conn Med.* 1985;49:805-819.

7. Horty J, Barker M. Provisional conduct. In: *Medical Staff Leader Handbook.* Pittsburgh: Action Kit Publications; 1999:1-38.

8. Gabbard G, Nadelson C. Professional boundaries in the physician-patient relationship. *JAMA.* 1996;273:1445-1449.

9. Gutheil TG, Gabbard G. Misuses and misunderstanding of boundary theory in clinical and regulatory settings. *Am J Psychiatry.* 1998;155:409-414.

10. Campbell M. The oath: an investigation of the injunction prohibiting physician-patient sexual relations. *Perspect Biol Med.* 1989;32:300-308.

11. Burgess AW. Physician sexual misconduct and patients' responses. *Am J Psychiatry.* 1981;138:1335-1342.

12. Feldman-Sommers S, Jones G. Psychological impacts of sexual contact between therapists or other health care practitioners and their clients. *J Consult Clin Psychol.* 1984;52:1054-1061.

13. Council on Ethical and Judicial Affairs, American Medical Association. Sexual misconduct in the practice of medicine. *JAMA.* 1991;266: 2741-2745.

14. American Psychiatric Association. *The Principles of Medical Ethics, with Annotations Especially Applicable to Psychiatry.* Washington, DC: American Psychiatric Press; 1995.

15. Medical Council of New Zealand. Sexual abuse in the doctor-patient relationship: discussion document for the profession. *Newslett Med Council N Z.* 1992;6:4-5.

16. Colorado Revised Statutes. The Medical Practice Act including 1995 amendments. Sections 12-36-117 (unprofessional conduct).

17. Simon RI. Sexual exploitation of patients: how it begins before it happens. *Psychiatr Ann.* 1989;9:104-112.

18. Epstein RS, Simon RI. The exploitation index: an early warning indicator of boundary violations in psychotherapy. *Bull Menninger Clin.* 1990;54:450-465.

19. Frick DE. Nonsexual boundary violations in psychiatric treatment. Im: Oldham JM, Reba MB, eds. *American Psychiatric Press Review of Psychiatry*. Washington, DC: American Psychiatric Press; 1994;13:415-432.

20. Gabbard G. Sexual misconduct. In: Oldham JM, Ruba MB, eds. *American Psychiatric Press Review of Psychiatry*. Washington, DC: American Psychiatric Press; 1994;13:488-456.

21. Waldinger RJ. Boundary crossings and boundary violations: thoughts on navigating a slippery slope. *Harvard Rev Psychiatry* 1994;2:225-227.

22. Gutheil TG, Gabbard G. The concept of boundaries in clinical practice: theoretical and risk-management dimensions. *Am J Psychiatry*. 1993;150:188-196.

23. Enbom JA, Thomas CD. Evaluation of sexual misconduct complaints: the Oregon board of medical examiners, 1991 to 1995. *Am J Obstet Gynecol*. 1997;176:1340-1348.

24. Dehlendorf CE, Wolfe SM. Physicians disciplined for sex-related offenses. *JAMA*. 1998;279:1883-1888.

25. Morrison J, Wickersham P. Physicians disciplined by a state medical board. *JAMA*. 1998;279:1889-1893.

26. Gabbard G. Psychodynamics of sexual boundary violations. *Psychiatr Ann*. 1991:21:651-655.

27. Irons R. On seduction and exploitation: a medical model approach. *Rhode Island Med*. 1994;77:354-356.

28. Schoener GR. Assessment of professionals who have engaged in boundary violations. *Psychiatr Ann*. 1995;25:95-99.

29. Dilts SL, Gendel M, Lepoff R, Clark C, Radcliff S. The Colorado physician health program: observations at 7 years. *Am J Addict*. 1996;4:337-345.

30. Abel GG, Barrett DH, Gardos PS. Sexual misconduct by physicians. *J Med Assoc Ga*. 1992;81:237-246.

31. Duckworth KM, Kahn M, Gutheil TG. Roles, quandaries and remedies: teaching professional boundaries to medical students. *Harvard Rev Psychiatry*. 1994;2:214-221, 227.

Chapter 10

Medical Students and Residents: Issues and Needs

Leah J. Dickstein, MD

A pplications to medical school do not specifically request information concerning applicants' past or current mental health status. During highly prized interviews, students do not usually offer, nor do interviewers ask for, such information. The same situation exists for the residents' application process. However, in my more than two decades of primary professional responsibility for mental health services for medical students and residents, issues of acute and chronic mental illness are rather common. Decades ago, one author stated that if adequate mental health services were available, as many as 65% of students would take advantage of this health care opportunity. Proportionally, women students and residents tend to seek outpatient services more readily, paralleling the general population. With time commitments often greater, residents are less likely to request services except for a major emergency in which symptoms interfere with their ability to function or they are referred for evaluation because of problems observed by others.

This chapter will discuss some of the barriers to the receiving of care by trainees and then go on to discuss discrete psychiatric disorders, specific stresses, and issues for particular trainee populations. Throughout the chapter, resident trainees will also be referred to as "students."

Barriers to Accepting and Accessing Help

Students ranked in the top and bottom quarters of their class are more likely than others to seek treatment. A significant number have been in therapy, counseling, or treatment before but intentionally did not make this known on their applications or in their interviews. Major concern and even fear about lack of confidentiality of their records and information too often bring them to therapy late. Their experiences in overhearing physicians, peers, and other health professionals glibly and carelessly talk about patients' problems, sometimes even worse, with inappropriate humor, in the physicians' lounge, hallways, elevators, or at the nurses' station heighten their hesitancy to seek consultation for evaluation. Beyond the fear of being talked and gossiped about, realistically they worry about the confidentiality of their medical records. Students are concerned about making and taking the time away from studying or missing classes, clinics, or rounds. They also worry about the confidentiality of their psychiatric/counseling records: who will have access to them now and later; how will their seeking treatment affect their later obtaining a medical license; what will be the impact on getting health and life insurance? All of these concerns are legitimate and must be discussed early and honestly with students.

The overriding issue of stigma, ie, becoming and being a psychiatric patient, must be raised and discussed repeatedly. If a school includes discussion of health care services and options in the admissions and recruitment materials and during orientation, students will be less loath to confront their personal mental illness and emotional problems. This direct inclusion of mental health needs can possibly decrease the stigma of mental illness and sometimes be lifesaving.

For example, at the University of Louisville, during a voluntary health promotion and prevention program, the Health Awareness Workshop, a panel of students discusses mental health issues of and for students, including their own hesitancies about acknowledging needs, trust in the school psychiatrists, and benefits of early intervention and appropriate treatment. The students' presentation often brings entering students to seek treatment much earlier, even during the four-day program, when they may reveal history of treatment or ongoing symptoms or simply seek reassurance that if their symptoms recur they can enter treatment easily.

The stigma of mental illness for medical students can be even more of a burden than for others. Some feel, "How can I be a competent student and then physician and simultaneously be a psychiatric patient?" Additionally, some share family histories of mental illness with an acknowledged shame, despite their knowledge of the genetics and neurobiology involved. Furthermore, there are other students who, when questioned, know of no relevant family history, yet when asked to discuss the issue with family members, return astonished (and often with visible relief), reporting that there is indeed a history of mental illness.

Another important issue related to stigma that must be raised early in any evaluation and treatment is the prognosis for most of the chief complaints students will present, mainly those of anxiety and depressive disorders. Many fear their symptoms represent an unending illness unique to them with only increased future disability to which they must look forward.

Ideally, there should be available to trainees an array of competent general medical and mental health professionals from whom the student or resident can elect to receive needed help. This will depend on many factors, including the availability of programs and professionals, a school's commitment of funds, insurance, and the accessibility of community professionals familiar with the unique problems of this population. Professionals selected to treat students and residents must be well trained, committed to their potential patients, and not overwhelmed by their issues or their academic accomplishments. Depending on the student's needs, the treatment type can be individual, dyadic (couple), family, or group. Psychodynamic, cognitive-behavioral, interpersonal, or systems approaches may be optimal.

Therapeutic involvement with the trainee's significant others, including parents, siblings, partner, children, or even grandparents, can at times be most helpful. Issues from the past or present can thus be corroborated and/or confronted. Furthermore, relationship issues can be discussed directly as the therapist observes the interactions. Long-held secrets of the student or the significant other (eg, sexual orientation, infidelity, abortion, adoption, etc) can be brought out safely and productively in a therapeutic setting. Of course, discussion beforehand as to what the student or resident wants to reveal or discuss is vital. The therapist should not be the messenger, but rather the trained listener, translator, and trusted support.

Discrete Psychiatric Disorders

As with the assessment of all psychiatric symptoms, a careful general medical and psychiatric history must be obtained, including a personal and three-generation biological family history. Students should be evaluated by their primary care physician (and encouraged to obtain one if they have not already done so). A physical exam, including a careful mental status exam, is critical. Depending on these findings, laboratory investigations may need to include complete blood cell count, urinalysis, toxicology for illicit drugs, chemistry profile, sedimentation rate, thyrotropin level, pregnancy test, B_{12} level, rapid plasma reagin/fluorescent treponemal antibody test, HIV test, and/or an electrocardiogram.

Alcohol and Other Substance Abuse

Alcohol and other substance abuse, including that of marijuana, opiates, benzodiazepines, and cocaine, continues to be a major health problem among trainees. Assessment and treatment issues are covered extensively in Chapter 8. The education of students and trainees at separate health promotion programs and at resident orientations should include this topic. Many schools or programs invite a physician from their state physician health program to speak to groups of trainees. In addition to offering a didactic presentation, this physician will often discuss his/her own recovery or bring along one or more physicians in recovery in his/her program to do so. If significant others of the trainees are also invited, they may learn about the early signs and symptoms of addiction and have a contact person and telephone number if problems arise later with their trainee-partner. This may allow for an earlier and perhaps even lifesaving intervention.

Depressive Disorders

Depressive disorders may be seen as:

- recurrent or first episodes of unipolar major depression
- secondary to or concurrent with other psychiatric illnesses (eg, an anxiety or substance use disorder)
- seasonal affective disorder
- dysthymic disorder
- bipolar depressive disorder (type I or II, or with mixed features)
- an early presentation of schizophrenia or schizoaffective disorder (both of which are rare in this group)

The treatment approaches may differ significantly among these various categories, so attention needs to be paid to proper diagnosis. It is also important to recognize when depression occurs secondary to a general medical condition or another psychiatric disorder, as treatment of the primary condition may improve the depression as well.

Suicide

Unfortunately, suicides among students and residents continue to occur. The risk of suicide needs to be considered and assessed as part of an evaluation for depressive and anxiety symptoms, psychotic symptoms (eg, in mania, depression, or schizophrenia), posttraumatic stress disorder (PTSD), and borderline personality disorder. Students must be asked about suicide thoughts; plans; and attempts, whether remote, repeated, or current. In addition, a family history of suicide should be obtained. Questioning a student about suicidal feelings or plans must always include asking about methods, including pills, firearms, and substances of abuse. Several nationally known student and resident suicides have included first the drinking of a large amount of alcohol followed by a fatal gunshot, jump, or overdose of other licit medications or illicit drugs.

Everyone involved in the teaching of students, including administration staff, must be aware of blatant dangerous behaviors and report them to the appropriate professional rather than turning away from ill students. This message must be delivered from and to the highest to the least senior levels of academic health center employees. Student suicides may occur at stressful academic and professional periods; after failing an exam; after a patient dies or an error is made in care; after a personal rejection in a relationship; following parents' unexpected divorce; or when there are legal problems of the student or a family member.

The overriding issue related to suicide by students and residents is that those around them ignore what they see and hear because of the "lonely pedestal" upon which these students and residents are placed, together with the denial and myriad of defenses used by these intelligent young professionals, who unfortunately end up tragically outsmarting themselves through their deaths. While many may voice aloud their frustrations, most don't intend to harm themselves, ie, "if I have one more assignment, or exam to prepare for, it's all over." Generally, those who complete suicide are silent rather than vocal, but by their changed behaviors may alert those around them. This requires being observant of another's personal pain and being strong enough to confront the student or resident observed to be on the edge of leaving life, or seeking others more appropriate or competent to manage the situation.

Anxiety Disorders

Anxiety disorders are the most common group of psychiatric illnesses among students and residents, just as they are among the general population. These include the following:

- generalized anxiety disorder
- panic disorder with agoraphobia (more common among women)
- specific and social phobias (the latter experienced, for example, by medical students having to present on ward rounds)

- the spectrum of PTSD symptoms, often resulting from victimization during childhood (child abuse) or in current relationships (intimate partner violence)

- obsessive-compulsive disorder, which may take the form of excessive handwashing (eg, after procedures or touching patients) or repeated checking of a patient's history or of facts about a disorder

A history of attempts at self-therapy for anxiety should be obtained, especially concerning the use or abuse of alcohol, marijuana, opiates, or benzodiazepines. Residents may write prescriptions for nonexistent patients, and students may also steal medications from wards and clinics or forge an attending's signature out of desperation (either to relieve anxiety or to block withdrawal symptoms).

Attention Deficit Hyperactivity Disorder

Attention deficit hyperactivity disorder (ADHD) is another problem for which students and residents seek treatment. They may have known they have this disorder for many years, have been in treatment, and have been taking medication but didn't want their school or department to know. Equally frequent is the situation where increased academic pressure prompts an evaluation for any learning disabilities, and the ADHD is first appreciated. There may be a strong sense of relief as they finally have an explanation for their previous occasional academic difficulties and "odd" behaviors that had seemed so mysterious. The response of the ADHD to medication and other treatments in adulthood is generally quite favorable.

Personality Disorders

Personality disorders are often missed in these young professionals. Antisocial behaviors and unexpected dependent behaviors in the men, particularly when they are rejected in personal relationships, should be identified. An unfortunate and generally unexpected behavior is cheating. This behavior has been found to be rampant among the brightest college students nationally, so it should perhaps not be too unexpected when some students revert to this practice later in their professional lives.

When borderline personality disorder appears to best describe presenting symptoms, generally in women, physicians must take the time to discern whether these behaviors may in part be symptoms of PTSD consequent to past and/or current abuse that the woman may have forgotten to mention, has repressed, or is fearful to divulge. Students with these problems must be assessed thoroughly and referred to those with particular expertise in this area.

Eating Disorders

Eating disorders are not uncommon among medical students. Although anorexia generally begins in early adolescence, many women students—often in the top of the class ranks—continue to suffer from this disorder well into young adulthood. Anorectic behavior may be coupled with bulimic bingeing and purging in a maladaptive attempt to cope with the distress felt from school or other pressures. Loose and layered clothing in the preclinical years should not be ignored, as it may represent a signal to such problems. These women— along with a smaller number of men (frequently gay-identified or denied)—may continue to excuse their thin appearances initially, or they may dissimulate about eating habits until confronted repeatedly in a supportive manner. Their relief is always evident when the truth is finally out. When the behaviors are disclosed, careful general medical and psychiatric histories and exams must be performed because of the medical morbidity and mortality associated with anorexia nervosa.

Insomnia

Insomnia is a common symptom, the cause of which is often misidentified by students. As a sole symptom, caffeine should rank high on the list of causal factors: more than 450 mg per day is itself considered caffeinism. A 12-ounce soft drink can contain 80 to 100 mg of caffeine, while regular drip coffee contains 80 to 120 mg (somewhat less in perked and instant). Alcohol typically disrupts sleep later in the night after its initial soporific effects have worn off. Nicotine too is a stimulant. Other agents that can also be implicated are over-the-counter drugs (eg, decongestants) and herbs and other naturopathic but nonregulated substances (eg, ephedra). Clearly, fear, anxiety, depression, or mild hypomania may also be implicated.

Body Dysmorphic Disorder

This is another psychiatric disorder that has an onset in this age group and that is frequently kept secret. Dermatologists, plastic surgeons, and primary care physicians in particular should be alert for students who seem unduly preoccupied with their physical appearance, especially if requests for cosmetic procedures are not consistent with the objective physiognomy.

Dissociative Identity Disorder

Dissociative identity disorder and other dissociative disorders are rare in the general population and likely rare but not absent among students. Those who have been severely abused (whether physically, sexually, or neglectfully) as children may have coped until, as young adults, they feel they can no longer do so. They may describe the experiences of "losing time," "running away in my mind," or "giving time to another part of me better able to handle it." With accurate diagnosis and competent psychotherapy, the prognosis is very good, and the student can expect that the disorder will not interfere with professional or personal goals.

Particular Stresses of Trainees

A useful way to think about students' stresses or problems is to separate them into two groups, those that they have in common with many young adults and those that are more unique to medical students and residents.

Adjustment Problems

Adjustment problems are common as students adapt to a new city, school/hospital, and/or living situation. Students often find themselves living alone and independently for the first time ever. Many have never shopped for food and cooked for themselves, especially in healthy ways. They are justifiably concerned about learning all the assigned material. They can be told that it is not necessarily more difficult but that the volume to be learned per unit of time may be at least twice that to which they are accustomed. Loneliness, inadequate study skills, academic pressures from within and without, or a first-ever exam failure can evolve into unease and a severe adjustment disorder.

Relationship Problems

Relationship problems are among the most common presenting complaints by students and residents. These may include:

- partner frustration because of the trainee's enormous time commitment to the profession
- infidelity by either partner despite academic and work responsibilities
- unexpected pregnancies
- unresolved anger over unbalanced responsibilities
- "the pedestal effect," ie, where the student/resident is treated as a special person because he/she is/will be a physician and therefore considers him or herself above normal responsibilities and respect for his or her partner

Too frequently, training obligations may be used as an excuse for not working on a relationship and for expecting "special privileges." At times the nonmedical partner is jealous, feeling or being made to feel inferior and at the beck and call of the student. Another all too common scenario is that of the "*duel*-career" couple, where verbal and nonverbal aggression, rather than discussion and negotiation by the dual-career couple, are the primary methods of communication. Relationship problems are discussed in greater detail in Chapter 5.

Unresolved Grief

For competent young professionals, a major personal and life stage issue may be that of unresolved personal grief over earlier life experiences. Although these students are so adept at using intellectualizing defenses, particularly suppression, the bubble eventually bursts, and they finally can no longer deny the pain of these personal events. Common examples include:

- having been given up for adoption and now needing to know the circumstances and reasons and to find their biologic parents

- having had an elective abortion: this experience may remain a major memory not only for women, but also for male partners, particularly when they were not part of the decision-making process

- parental separations, divorces, remarriages, affairs and deaths: despite current adult status and academic competencies, often these students continue to carry the belief that they could or should have done something to prevent the catastrophe. Often, their presenting complaint centers around a thought such as, "I can't continue feeling guilty if I call my Dad because then I'm not being supportive of my mother after all that happened."

- awareness that they have brought learned dysfunctional personal behaviors to current relationships and finding that their personal relationships mimic those that they observed in their unhappy homes growing up

Dysfunctional Family Legacies

An inordinate number of those entering medicine come with experiences beginning in childhood of having been cast in the long-running role of *family helpers or rescuers.* This may stem from having had one or both parents with their own medical, psychiatric, and/or substance abuse problems. In current relationships, the students are likely to be repeating their rescuer roles. This inappropriate role and its consequent power imbalance can bring confused and unhappy students to seek help.

In a similar vein, residual effects of childhood family violence for students are not uncommon. Physical, sexual, verbal, or psychological abuse can take their toll many years later. Gender differences are seen, as there has been a greater likelihood of sexual abuse of the women and more physical abuse of the men. Adult problem behaviors may include suicide attempts, intimate partner violence, or even stalking of peers by the student/resident.

Adult children of alcoholics typically face a number of issues from their troubled childhoods, and they may wish to avail themselves of groups that are often available within the university, or even the academic health center itself.

Chronic Medical Illnesses

Chronic medical illnesses also occur in some of the students. Among the more common conditions seen in this age group are Crohn's disease, ulcerative colitis, irritable bowel disease, multiple sclerosis, myasthenia gravis, rheumatoid arthritis, and essential hypertension. Certain malignancies, such as Hodgkin's disease and testicular cancer, are among the more common cancers seen in young adults, and their diagnosis may precipitate an emotional crisis. Yet, with good medical care, a positive attitude, family and significant-other support, and attention to the psychosocial aspects of care, students can deal with these chronic illnesses. Some students evince an interest in complementary medicine to accompany more traditional medical care: relaxation techniques such as meditation, t'ai chi, and music may be helpful in managing the anxiety that may accompany illness. The effects of disabilities on trainees and tools to accommodate them are discussed in Chapter 3.

HIV/AIDS Testing

Not surprisingly, HIV testing of students and residents is not an uncommon issue. Whether the student has had an inadvertent needle-stick or fears that a past or current sexual relationship may involve HIV infection, fear or terror is present, often followed by shame. Referral for expert medical evaluation should be made promptly, whether to infectious disease specialists or to a public health clinic (for anonymous testing). Supportive psychotherapy may be needed for such crises.

"I Don't Really Want to Be a Physician"

Several academically successful students annually seek consultation when they realize they can no longer contain this truth. Ashamed and guilty to have "wasted all these years and will now disappoint my parents and teachers," they then begin experiencing somatic symptoms of anxiety and depression, together with self-isolation and fear they "never will be happy." With psychotherapeutic work they can usually decide if these feelings are primary, or if they are secondary to other unrecognized issues. If primary, with support and planning they usually leave medicine and enter a field in which they will be able both to earn a living and to find personal contentment. If secondary, they may come to recognize the source of their doubts and alleviate them.

Issues for Particular Trainee Populations

Women

Too often, women medical students find themselves assuming impossible superwoman roles and come for help believing they are simply inadequate. Other women seek understanding and treatment because they find the personal loneliness and difficulties in meeting a partner overwhelming. Despite the changing and enlarged expectations and possibilities for women in work and personal roles in society at large, it is still too often the norm in many medical training cultures that women are expected to remain confined to more stereotypic, limited roles. Some women in medical training feel more comfortable being more assertive at school and in the hospital, but not in their personal lives, and this can pose an ongoing, common difficulty. The reverse situation creates its own set of problems for women as well.

Women tend to bear most of the burden of abuses of power in medical settings. *Sexual harassment,* a particular type of abuse of power, continues at all levels of medical education and training, and it is primarily directed toward women and primarily engaged in by men. Typically, the male harassers are preclinical and clinical faculty and chief residents. However, not only are supervisors or teachers at all levels potential perpetrators, but patients and their visitors too may harass trainees.

Victims (primarily women, less often gay men, least frequently heterosexual men) often fear coming forward to report such unlawful behaviors in the belief that they will not be believed. Unfortunately, this may be realistic. The abusive behaviors and ways of communication seen in sexual harassment reflect societal stereotypes and can only be eliminated by ongoing directives from those in the most senior leadership roles. Thus, ongoing education of the entire medical school community, including hospital staff, must be mandatory. In addition, there must be clear roles for proper behavior and safe reporting, together with real repercussions for infractions. Everyone at the medical center must be taught that observers of sexual harassment—or any form of mistreatment or abuse—should report what they see as part of being a responsible member of the community. Posters in waiting rooms, restrooms, and elevators can constructively present the issue and help delineate correct rules of behavior and the consequences of noncompliance.

Men

Men too can become trapped by limiting stereotypes of gender roles. Though male students and residents may succeed academically and professionally, their emotional reactions to life events may remain more problematic. They may adhere to a gender stereotype of the "white knights," a false model of "men in white" who are invulnerable and strong, whether coping with feelings produced by patient encounters, by supervisors' evaluations, or in their personal lives. These men, particularly when they are rejected by an intimate partner, may become overwhelmed with feelings of helplessness. They may not recognize their normal feelings of dependency and vulnerability and become acutely, deeply distressed, even suicidal or homicidal. Immediate interventions are necessary to protect them from their suicidal or (less frequently) homicidal impulses. This would then be followed by psychotherapy (individually or in a group) to explore and modify the crippling effects of these stereotypes.

Homosexual Students

Gay, lesbian, and bisexual students often must face issues that come to the fore during school and training. Medical school and training years typically overlap the young adult developmental task of finally coming to terms with one's sexual identity. Students who had previously remained in the closet may feel a need to come out, not only to families, significant others, peers, and teachers, but often to themselves as well. Coming out—or remaining out if this had been done earlier in life—can be made more difficult by a medical center culture that is homophobic. Ongoing conflicts over sexual identity can definitely interfere in academic pursuits, so assistance needs to be provided, regardless of whether the source of the conflicts is internal or environmental.

Schools and hospitals can make available publicity about support groups in the community and within the medical centers where they exist. Membership in the American Medical Student Association's committee on gay/lesbian/bisexual issues and the Gay and Lesbian Medical Association can also offer students a support network. These groups can also assist those who are seeking professional help to work through their life experiences and feelings, including their own internalized homophobia, and to reach greater self-acceptance.

Ethnic Minorities

Racial discrimination is often an unexpected and potentially devastating experience for students and residents. Walking from the library to a preclinical class and being accosted by a public safety officer with the words, "What are you doing here," or being confronted in a similar fashion in a hospital corridor while rushing to obtain lab results without a white jacket are unfortunately not unheard-of occurrences for these trainees. Because they have been academically successful, some of these young adults may not have encountered much discrimination earlier in their lives, and the current experience becomes particularly unsettling. It is important that they be able to find and trust some staff, administrators, or faculty onsite to whom they can report and process this. Additionally, preorientation programs can bring together students from diverse backgrounds (not only racial/ethnic, but also sexual orientation and geographic) for presentations about diversity, raising issues and encouraging acceptance and inclusiveness by the entire community of students, faculty, and staff. These can be taught as important steps to building a healthy and caring student community.

Nontraditional Students

Second-career or nontraditional students may experience their own unique stressors. Having overcome years of preparation to enter medicine, often on a part-time basis while maintaining work and family responsibilities, they may find themselves having a harder time adjusting to academic demands. A first-ever F or being in the lowest class quartile for the first time may be devastating. This inferior academic record may raise questions in the student's mind as to whether he or she really belongs there, or whether he or she should continue despite years of dogged preparation.

Separation, divorce, remarriage, step-parenting, and single parenting are obviously more common in these students, and dealing with these issues can lead to requests for assistance. Maintaining full-time medical commitment while resolving these often unexpected issues can be daunting. Other problems more likely to be faced by these students include dependent care for children, children's illnesses or other immediate needs, infertility, and elderly relatives' dependent care needs.

The needs for prevention, health promotion, and early recognition and intervention programs are clear. I have developed an example of such a comprehensive set of programs, included in the Appendix.

Suggested Readings

Aach RD. Alcohol and other substance abuse and impairment among physicians in residency training. *Ann Intern Med.* 1992;116:245-254.

Baldwin DC, Hughes PH, Conard SE, et al. Substance abuse among senior medical students: a survey of 23 medical schools. *JAMA.* 1991;265:2074-2078.

Christie JD, Rosen IM, Bellini LM, et al. Prescription drug use and self-prescriptions among resident physicians. *JAMA.* 1998;280:1253-1255.

Clark DC, Zeldow PB. Vicissitudes of depressed mood during four years of medical school. *JAMA.* 1988;260:2521-2528.

Colford JM, McPhee SJ. The ravelled sleeve of care: managing the stresses of residency training. *JAMA.* 1989;261:889-893.

Dickstein LJ. *Health Awareness Workshop Reference Manual.* Louisville, KY: Proactive Press; 1998.

Dickstein LJ, Stephenson JJ, Hinz L. Psychiatric impairment in medical students. *Acad Med.* 1990;65:588-593.

Hays LR, Cheever T, Patel P. Medical student suicide, 1989-1994. *Am J Psychiatry.* 1995;153:553-555.

Hughes PH, Conard SE, Baldwin DC, et al. Resident physician substance use in the United States. *JAMA.* 1991;265:2069-2073.

Komaromy M, Bindman AB, Haber RJ. Sexual harassment in medical training. *N Engl J Med.* 1993;328:322-326.

Peterkin AD. *Staying Human During Residency Training.* Ottawa, ON: Canadian Medical Association; 1991.

Sheehan KH, Sheehan DV, White K, et al. A pilot study of medical student abuse: student perceptions of mistreatment and misconduct in medical school. *JAMA.* 1990;263:533-537.

Appendix

Description of the University of Louisville Medical Student Health Promotion and Prevention Programs

The Chief of Mental Health Services (the Chief) must be present at all mandatory student and resident orientation programs. This person, his/her title, office, telephone. and emergency numbers must be known and made available to all at the academic health center. The Chief must also attend all voluntary health promotion programs.

The *Health Awareness Workshop*, which began in 1981, is held four days before the mandatory orientation day. It is a support and prevention program for entering students and their significant others. About 40 second-year students voluntarily return one week early to shop and cook three healthy meals per day under the direction of a staff nutritionist in the Department of Family and Community Medicine; most meals are vegetarian. No caffeine or alcohol is served. Presentations, made every morning by university faculty, include the importance of health awareness, introduction to the medical school via its history, and the physiology and importance of exercise.

The class is assigned to one of six rooms, where they have desks, study carels, and computers. The 23 students in each room are assigned several second-year "health tutors"; other health tutors include a preclinical PhD, a clinical MD, and a resident. This team meets with their unit lab the first through the fourth day for lunch. This is an opportunity for introductions and for upperclass students, faculty, and the resident to offer healthy advice, for school tours, blood pressure, height, and weight measurements and the opportunity to begin to get to know classmates. This same support team will continue to meet with the first-year students during the school year as "The Student Hour."

The *SOUL (Student Outreach at the University of Louisville)* is another support program. Up to five students from each class are selected to be available to any students who seek assistance. Phone numbers and other methods of contact are noted on a SOUL wallet card, with voluntary community physicians, faculty physicians (primarily not psychiatrists), several residents, the State Director of the Physicians Health Committee, and the Chief of Mental Health Services.

The *Advocates* program is another support system. For each unit lab of 23 first-year students, there are two second-year Advocates who must check on their charges at least four of five days weekly; observe changes, absences, and disturbances; and, when necessary, contact a qualified administrator (Associate Dean for Faculty and Student Advocacy, the Associate Dean for Student Affairs, the Chief of Mental Health Services, and any other person unique to that school).

Several *publications* are part of the program. The Health Awareness Newsletter is a monthly two-page collection of health tips, students' poetry, special events, and an editor's column by the Associate Dean for Faculty and Student Advocacy. There are handouts during the Health Awareness Workshop, in particular a 127-page handbook of useful information beyond coping with academics, for personal health and impairment issues. There is a Substance Abuse Library Resource Center with books and films in the Advocacy Office. Offering students and residents easy unquestioned access to these materials, the total list is given to each student during the Health Awareness Workshop, where it may eventually be the first step in giving the student the courage to seek treatment.

There are ongoing presentations to all faculty at department meetings discussing *sexual harassment and medical student abuse* to raise awareness and encourage appropriate behaviors on the part of all, especially those with power, and therefore with the power to abuse power, as well as the power to stop abuse of students and residents being perpetrated by others.

Each school and academic health center must ensure that there is a variety of publicized support and intervention programs available to all students and residents.

Meeting former student and resident physicians years later at professional meetings, or hearing from them and learning of lives filled with personal happiness and contentment and abilities to meet life's personal challenges, in addition to valued contributions to medicine in all its possible practice forms, is sufficient and clear evidence that we must be responsive and responsible to our young students and trainees at one of their most vulnerable life stages. Clearly, it is well worth our efforts and a reflection of all the oaths we take as physicians to serve our peers and patients ethically and well.

Chapter 11

The Aging Physician

Marion Zucker Goldstein, MD

Accoding to the 1997-1998 edition of the American Medical Association's *Physician Characteristics and Distribution in the US*, the "aging" (age 65 years and over) physician population is 125,162, or 17.0% of a total physician population of 737,764. In the 1999 edition of this reference, an additional 18,946 physicians are reported in the total number. Overall, the rate of increase of physician growth has been four times faster than that of the general population during the past 36 years. These figures highlight that the number of older physicians is already sizable and also is growing rapidly.

By comparison, those aged 65 years and over constitute on average between 12% and 16% (depending on geographic region) of the general population, with considerably more women than men with each advancing decade. The group of physicians aged 65 years and over, however, contrasts with this gender ratio. Some 114,792 (19.0%) of a total of 580,377 male physicians were aged 65 years and over, while 10,370 (15.0%) out of a total of 157,387 women physicians were aged 65 years and over. This group includes 55,952 (48.7%) of the total of 114,792 male physicians who are listed as "inactive" compared to 5,342 women (51.5%) of the 10,370 aged 65 years and over. In the group 55 to 64 years of age, there are 99,498 total physicians, 88,665 men and 10,833 (10.9%) women. Eighteen percent of men and 10% of women in the 55- to 64-year-old group reported being inactive. Breakdown by decade of the total number of physicians aged 65 years and over who reported being professionally inactive is not available. Figure 11-1 summarizes some of these data.

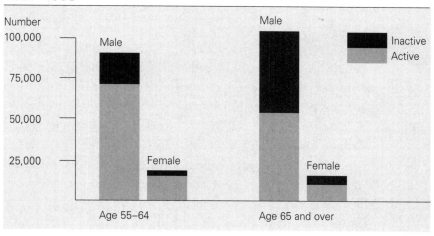

From 1970 to 1996, the male-to-female ratio in the group aged 65 years and over did not change and remained at 92% men to 8% women. During this same period, there were noteworthy increases in total number of male physicians (from 334,028 to 737,764), in number of female physicians (from 25,401 to 157,387) and in international medical graduates (IMGs), (from 57,217 to 169,826). The number of female IMG physicians rose most dramatically during the past two decades. The IMG group accounted for 23% of the total physician population, and 14.3% within this group were aged 65 years and over in 1996. In 1970, 58.4% of women physicians were under 45 years old, with a rise to 67.5% by 1996, reflecting a sixfold absolute increase in numbers overall. In other words, the current older physician population does not reflect the demographic changes seen in the overall physician population during the past 25 years.

Race/ethnicity is known for only 64% of physicians, with their distribution in 37 specialties. Whites account for 80%, blacks for 3%, Hispanics for 5%, Asian/Orientals for 10%, and others for the remainder. More accurate and detailed distributions, especially for diversity of ethnic presence among the 65-and-over group of physicians, may have to be obtained from specialty organizations. Fear that knowledge of ethnicity will lead to prejudice and discrimination rather than improved cultural training, knowledge, understanding, and accommodation continues to create difficulties in getting this information.

Female physicians have suffered from a severe lack of role models and the lack of advantage possessed by many male colleagues who had wives at home to tend to their personal, office management, and/or families' needs. This has contributed to varying degrees of excess stress and compromised personal and professional lifestyles for this group of older women who entered the medical profession. On the other hand, they have greatly benefitted from organized and informal supports they could give to each other, which was considerably more difficult to establish for the 8% of women physicians in the 65-and-over group. Attitudes of some younger men have changed, and some are now more willing and eager to be partners at home.

The group of physicians aged 65 years and over graduated from medical school four or more decades ago. Many became general practitioners (41.9%), compared to 6.0% among primary care physicians of all ages in 1995. Others did residencies in various specialties. Older female physicians are primarily represented (1,000 or more) in seven specialties, whereas the younger group is represented in 17 specialties. Those physicians who chose an academic career had mostly male mentors, and many men rose in the ranks and became tenured professors in medical schools. Major professional activities are not listed by age and gender; however, more than 80% of both IMGs and women list "patient care" as their primary activity, and more men have other professional activities such as administration, teaching, and research. The marked underrepresentation of women in administration (more authority and higher salaries) and as professors in medical schools is well documented and is particularly apparent in the 65-and-over group.

Relatively little research is available as to what contributes to professional inactivity with age among physicians or, conversely, what factors lead physicians who remain professionally active to an advanced age to do so. A vast variety of professional activities and specialties, family constellations, other interests and commitments, and work environments in the current health care system make any attempt at generalization about the aging physician's profile an oversimplification that needs to be modified by individualization for person and situation. The elderly, including elderly physicians, are a very heterogeneous group in our population.

Physicians' Planning for Their Own Aging

Though many of their patients live to ever more advanced years, physicians, except for those who have acquired special knowledge and competence in geriatric medicine, geriatric psychiatry, or geriatric family practice, seldom pay much attention to age-linked manifestations, vulnerabilities, potential preventive measures, or age-appropriate assessments and treatments. Research has shown that physicians as a group do not abide by their own advice to patients in terms of healthy lifestyle (including physical fitness and nutrition) and regular medical attention and workup. Many do not attend to interventions that could delay or alleviate age-related decline in cognition, mobility, sensory acuities, and functions of various organ systems.

Inadequate understanding and knowledge of aging processes leads to lack of attention to the need to adapt gradually to changes with age and to make gradual preparations for retirement. Thus, when acute or chronic disease strikes, abrupt retirement or partial retirement becomes more likely and may create additional emotional and financial hardships. In addition, in many places health care services for the elderly, including the elderly physician, remain fragmented and difficult to access, with too few trained physicians to give adequate treatment, too few specialty-trained physicians to refer to, and ongoing discriminatory reimbursement for mental health care.

With often ample incomes from busy practices, physicians frequently have paid little attention to effective financial planning for retirement. Long hours and stressful clinical and administrative responsibilities are additional factors constraining financial, health, and recreational planning for retirement by the aging physician. Changes in the health care delivery system—and their many growing burdens on physicians—have led to an increase in early retirements, regardless of discipline, competence, or physical or mental state of the physician. Some physicians have switched to nonclinical health care positions, have developed diversified sources of income, or have shifted to nonmedical careers altogether. However, opportunities to undertake such changes are undesirable to some and not available to others in later life.

In general, the older physician is more likely to resist the need for improved strategies and tools for managing information, measuring outcomes, reducing costs, and improving quality under rapidly changing circumstances, or to accept mandates to enhance efficiency and profitability. Considerable new learning and time commitments are required, which he or she may not have much time left to apply and from which to benefit. Chapter 14 discusses many of these career issues in greater detail.

Potential Effects of Aging on Clinical Competence

Self-awareness is key to adaptation to aging, since everyone ages differently and different manifestations can occur at different ages. Common manifestations of several aging organ systems will be reviewed here.

Vision

The following components of vision frequently diminish gradually with advancing age:

- visual acuity
- depth perception
- night vision (lengthened dark-adaptation time, increased glare sensitivity)
- color discrimination
- range of visual fields

If ophthalmologic corrections are no longer effective, these visual changes slow down reaction time; diminish precision; and can affect driving, surgical performance, and execution of other procedures that require eye-hand coordination. These changes in vision can contribute to misinterpretations of pathology projected on screens and radiologic and ultrasound readings.

Psychomotor

With aging, motor response time lengthens, manual dexterity diminishes, and tremors are more common and will ultimately affect performance despite speed attained with repetitive practice over the years. Complex cases and situations and the learning of new technologies and new concepts need to be given more time because they become more difficult to master in later life than they are for most younger physicians.

Hearing

Auditory deficits develop in about 24% of persons between the ages of 65 and 74 years. Even if optimally corrected, this condition can contribute to misunderstandings and delays in responsiveness.

Cognition

Age may limit cognitive abilities such as:

- ability to focus attention
- sustaining concentration over long periods of time
- selectively attending to the most important stimulus out of many
- accomplishing multifactorial tasks simultaneously
- learning new and unfamiliar material in a short period of time
- immediate memory and recall

Though overall IQ declines with aging, usually creativity and scientific output do not. The natural slowing seems to provide more time for creative expression if such opportunities remain, are made available, or are actively sought out. The many frustrating situations brought about by increased impairment of immediate memory and delayed recall can only be reduced in frequency and intensity by adaptive slowing. They can also be ameliorated by the companionship and working relationships with younger friends, colleagues, and family who are as yet unencumbered by these manifestations and are able and willing to "fill in." Searching for words and names and misplacing items of everyday use become more frequent, and time spent in retrieval and recall becomes longer.

Sleep and Sex

Sleeping patterns and sexual patterns change during the aging process. "Routines" from previous years may become inappropriate, and rescheduling professional and personal activities during high-energy times of the day and rest periods at other times of the day becomes highly desirable for ongoing satisfaction, productivity, and enjoyment.

Age-related Illnesses

Various diseases occur and need to be dealt with more frequently in later life than earlier in life. Cataracts and glaucoma become more common after age 65 years. Limitation of motion and pain caused by arthritis occurs in nearly half the population after age 65 years. Balance diminishes, falls are more frequent, and the consequences are more severe. Osteoporosis, especially in women, predisposes to back pain and vertebral, hip, and other fractures. Healing takes longer. Cardiac disease, vascular disease, and cancer take their toll, as do dementia, parkinsonism, depression, anxiety, delirium, and other neuropsychiatric disorders. Increased sensitivity to prescribed and over-the-counter medications and alcohol secondary to changing functions in various organ systems—hepatic, renal, gastrointestinal, gonadal, central nervous system, musculoskeletal, endocrine, immune—has to be taken into account. The body's fat and water distribution changes, increasing the way some medications are distributed and accumulate in the body.

Adapting to Changes

Providers of health care need to modify their practices according to the aging processes in their elderly patients, be they physiologic or pathologic. All older patients, including older physicians as patients, need to become active partners in this communication and practice modification by volunteering information and observations related to aging. Physicians need to learn to listen and assist in the process of aging and its vicissitudes, which includes enduring and adapting to losses in health, relationships, and familiar environments. Depression and anxiety experienced secondary to perceiving age-related manifestations as "loss" of youthful ideals only stand in the way of adaptation and, if present, need to be attended to by appropriate mental health interventions.

A gradual change from a life committed to physicianhood, patient care with or without teaching, research, and administration of one kind or other is more likely to be rewarding and successful than sudden change. Preparation for the future by developing interests and skills earlier in life outside of professional training can lead to fulfillment in later life. Involvement and engagement in many aspect of life, including physical fitness, healthy nutrition, health and mental health care, socialization, spiritual observance or involvements, an intimate other, and the rewards of lifelong money management, can contribute to well-being in retirement. The myth that physicians do not get ill and do not require the supports they are expected to deliver to others needs to be refuted by physicians and others alike.

Retirement Planning and Experiences

Many salaried physicians have pension plans and are offered retirement incentives without having an obligatory retirement age, compared to those who have practiced independently in the United States. Older physicians who have practiced independently may over time lose equity in their practice, may not be able to retire for financial reasons, or may not be able to work part-time because of high overhead and loss of value of their practice.

The Canadian government in various provinces is working on retirement packages to help physicians retire, such as opportunities to sell billing numbers back to the province to help cover practice closing costs. Government pension plans are being considered in various provinces, and the Canadian Medical Association's MD Management Division, which handles financial planning for physicians, reports that a growing number of medical students and residents are seeking advice and more younger physicians are attending retirement workshops. Conflicts have arisen over policies for reduced fees for new physicians instead of buyout programs for older doctors and lack of long-term planning for the careers of physicians that includes dignified retirement without financial catastrophe for young or old, opportunities for practice for new generalists and specialists, and timely quality delivery of medical care to the population. With mandatory retirement for all physicians at age 70 years, by 2005 each physician would serve about 787 people in Canada, and with required retirement at 65 years the number would be 847, if emigration of 800 physicians annually is included in these calculations. In the United States, there are 282 physicians per 100,000 population, or about one physician per 498 people.

In the United States, studies of retiring and retired physicians have been undertaken in several states. In Minnesota, a survey of all retired physicians revealed that 73% retired in their 60s and 22% at 65. Good health was reported by 69%; 64% reported comfortable incomes and 14% stated that income was barely adequate. The study showed that retired physicians considered nonmedical activities much more important than medical activities. These activities included visiting family (86%), reading (79%), and travel (63%). A California study of retired physicians living in Los Angeles County showed similar findings and, in addition, found that health often improved after retirement, as did relationships with spouse and children. Retired physicians engaged in a wide range of interests and activities. Emotional difficulties were reported as considerably *reduced* after retirement.

An Australian study compared retired psychiatrists with working psychiatrists. Significant differences were found in that almost 50% of *working* psychiatrists aged 55 years and over had reduced their hours in the previous five years; 61% were in private practice, whereas 53% of the *retired* group had been in the public sector. Of note was that significantly more *working* psychiatrists anticipated deteriorating health and family/personal problems as reasons for retiring and anticipated considerably more postretirement professional activities than *retired* psychiatrists were actually involved in.

Retirement from Academic Medicine

Observations in many academic environments show that retired chairs of departments, though they have given up administrative responsibilities, frequently maintain access to resources in the department such as space, secretarial help, and research assistance and contribute in manners of their choosing to research, teaching, and patient care. The established "buddy network" among deans and chairs, mostly men, is sustained with frequent national and international travel with wives. Women physicians in academia, unless married to men with prestige in the academic hierarchy, tend to be allotted fewer amenities in the system and tend to maintain more of the responsibilities from which they may wish to retire. Some examples of retirement behaviors of academic physicians follow.

- A past chairman of medicine became a consultant in a health maintenance organization and subsequently to its physician practice management company. He continued to write chapters, edit books, and serve on university committees. He would show up to meetings at his convenience and excuse himself gracefully when debates became repetitive and unproductive. He remained a major contributor, able to size up situations quickly and problem solve insightfully because "he had been there before."

- A woman professor continued in all activities after "retirement," maintained a prolific record of scientific publications with colleagues now as first author, developed and ran service programs, and gave lectures all over the country. She maintained contact with hundreds of colleagues and relatives regularly. She received many honors and awards. She only limited her traveling when her husband, a professor at the same institution, became seriously ill and needed a great deal of care. Being a grandmother became a significant part of her later life.

- A woman physician research scientist and professor in her late 60s continued to do research mainly funded by industry, no longer supported by renewable five-year federal grants that had kept her laboratory and staff going for many years. She remained on committees at the medical school and continued her rotation on service. Departmental secretarial assistance or research assistance had not been made available to her.

- A physician who had been a university professor for many years was offered a position at one of the major pharmaceutical companies as a consultant. This represented a new late-life challenge and a major relief to be a consultant for a wealthy part of the health care industry.

- Another professor gave up each of his three jobs that constituted his salary, one at a time, over the course of several years. Well respected locally, he focused his contributions on specialized services for the elderly in various settings and lectures in the community on occasion. He maintained modest administrative and service commitments. He had been ill on several occasions and assumed responsibilities for elderly ailing parents and in-laws together with his retired wife.

Retirement from Private Practice

Retiring from private practice solo, a small group, a large group, or a combination of jobs and private practice can often create a more abrupt change of identity and lifestyle. Though planning years in advance is recommended, once patients, staff, and overhead have been transferred or terminated and there is no reason to remain on a hospital staff, the daily routine of going to work has ended as has the physician identity. The emotional and physical reactions to loss of position, income, purpose, and stimulation of an active professional life all have to be gradually prepared for and actively replaced by other activities within or outside the medical arena.

Closing a practice is a complex matter and may occur for many different reasons. Specialists with no night call, no surgical responsibilities, and relatively low overhead (such as psychiatrists) have the oldest median retirement age.

Surgeons, despite the potentially detrimental effects of the aging process on performance and risk-benefit ratio for patients under their care, are a typical group of physicians for whom there are no institutionalized retirement criteria and who as a group pay little attention to the lifestyle they wish to establish after retirement. A survey of members of the American College of Surgeons revealed that only a small percentage of surgeons under age 70 years had a well-defined financial plan for their future. This has been considered to reflect many surgeons' difficulties in perceiving a life beyond surgery and the often single-minded dedication to their work at the expense of partaking in the richness of identity and life outside of their chosen field.

Because of the severe financial losses that can be incurred when closing a practice, it is important to do so in a timely, orderl, and well-thought-out fashion. The AMA has published a document entitled, "Closing Your Practice: 7 Steps to a Successful Transition," which explains many of they steps involved (see Chapter 15 for reference).

Retiring from partnerships can be planned gradually by hiring younger physicians to whom patients can be referred when the older partner is ready to diminish the volume and complexity of his/her practice and is willing to reduce personal income. Such gradual withdrawal can be worked out with legal and tax advice without jeopardizing the value of the overall practice he/she had either bought into or helped build many years ago and without jeopardizing the health and well-being of partners.

Having a postretirement plan within and outside the medical profession that includes dealing with personal and family health issues appears to make for the best adaptation after retirement. We have many years to plan and train for our careers and need as many years to plan for our retirement in sickness or health.

Suggested Readings

American Medical Association. *Closing Your Practice*. Chicago: American Medical Association; 1997.

American Medical Association. *Physician Characteristics and Distribution in the US, 1997-1998*. Chicago: American Medical Association; 1998.

Buske L. Projected physician supply. *Can Med Assoc J.* 1998;158:1584.

Dobrof R, Moody HR, Disch R, eds. *Dignity and Old Age*. New York: Haworth Press Inc; 1999.

Goldberg JH. Closing your practice, starting planning years ahead. *Med Econ.* 1994;71:151-160.

Goldberg JH. When or whether to retire. *Med Econ.* 1992;69:163-175.

Greenfield LZ, Proctor MC. When should a surgeon retire? *Adv Surg.* 1999;32:385-393.

Sanmartin CA, Snidal L. Profile of the Canadian physicians. *Can Med Assoc J.* 1993;149:971-984

Rowe JW, Kahn RL. *Successful Aging*. New York: Pantheon Books; 1998.

Sadavoy J Lazarus L, Jarvik LF, Grossbert G, ed. *Comprehensive Review of Geriatric Psychiatry II*. Washington, DC: American Psychiatric Press, Inc; 1996.

Weis SS, Kaplan EH, Flanagan CH. Aging and retirement: a difficult issue for individual psychoanalysts and organized psychoanalysis. *Bull Menninger Clin.* 1997;61:469-480.

Chapter 12

When Physicians Become Ill

Larry S. Goldman, MD

I t is a truth universally acknowledged that, as a group, physicians have a hard time becoming and being patients. The social roles assigned by society to the physician and to the patient are vastly different and at times appear almost incompatible. Many of the traits and skills that are most greatly valued by physicians can, unfortunately, be the ones that make being a patient unpleasant. The physician's needs to be in control and omniscient, not to be dependent on others, and to put aside his or her emotional reactions, for example, all render adaptation to the role of patient difficult. Add to this the strong underlying fear of illness and death that many physicians possess even before their medical training, and the transition from physician to patient becomes even more complicated.

This chapter is divided into two main sections. The first section discusses the course of the physician's experience with an illness: it explores the reaction to the possibility of illness (when symptoms occur), to getting medical help and obtaining a diagnosis, and then to coping with the illness itself. The second section covers the reactions of others—family members, colleagues, patients, and the workplace—to these events. Although these processes may at times go smoothly for all concerned, the chapter will emphasize common problems and pitfalls and some ways to prevent or minimize them. It is important to emphasize that there is no "typical" or "predictable" course that is taken, as the events and reactions are shaped by the physician's personality, the illness and illness course itself, and the physician's support system. In this way, of course, physician-patients are no different from any other patient.

Physician Reactions to Illness Course

Despite their intellectual ability to interpret symptoms that they develop, it is common for physicians to react to symptoms in ways that they would never suggest to others:

> **Case Vignette.** Dr R was a 62-year-old internationally respected academic general surgeon. Despite a family history of coronary artery disease, a significant personal smoking history, and a proudly flaunted "type triple A" personality, he regarded his frequent and worsening chest pains as bothersome indigestion or musculoskeletal problems, and he maintained his 14-hour clinical and teaching days seven days a week as he alternated between gulping anti-inflammatory and antacid medications. His denial was eventually pierced when he collapsed onto a patient in the operating room during a procedure and regained consciousness in the coronary care unit 12 hours after his cardiopulmonary resuscitation.

The Decision to Seek Care

There are a number of reasons that physicians may deny or minimize the import of symptoms they develop; these are summarized in Table 12-1. One set of reasons involves fears attendant on what will be discovered and what illness course might ensue. This is largely a function of having seen worst-case scenarios during training or practice, but it may be enhanced by preexisting hypochondriacal tendencies, counterphobic reactions to fears of illness,[*] or the pessimistic thinking seen sometimes in depression or dysthymia. Physicians may therefore think catastrophically about the meaning of symptoms, so that, for example, a nosebleed becomes equated with uncontrolled hypertension, a blood dyscrasia, or leukemia rather than simply a dried nasal lining from a low-humidity environment. Even if the illness threat seems manageable, there may be exaggerated fears of the diagnostic process or the treatments required. Physicians in general tend to overestimate the probabilities of adverse events, and this tendency is likely to increase in situations where they have a personal stake in the outcome.

---

[*] As noted in Chapters 2 and 4, many physicians enter medical training with exaggerated fears of illness or death, and their enthusiasm for medicine may represent a (counterphobic) method of dealing with these anxieties.

Table 12-1
Some Reasons that Physicians Deny or Minimize Symptoms

- Fear of what symptoms mean
- Fear of medical care mishaps
- Overvalued ability to self-diagnose
- Concerns over impact of illness on practice
- Difficulty entrusting care to colleagues
- Concerns over reactions of patients, colleagues, family
- Worries about confidentiality
- Avoidance of discomfort or indignities of diagnostic work-up or treatment

A second set of concerns has to do with interacting with the health care system in a different role from the usual. There may be issues having to do with privacy, confidentiality, and maintaining dignity. Just as physicians may catastrophize about their illness, they may also be concerned about the harm that may befall them from receiving care by exaggerating the likelihood and severity of potential medical errors or mishaps.

The third group of concerns relates to the physician's practice. There are often significant worries about how an illness would affect the perceptions of one's patients, colleagues, and others with whom the physician works. The fear is generally that one's worth will be seen as diminished by being ill or that others will feel that the physician is not carrying a fair share of the workload. Most physicians who become ill report that their patients are highly supportive, and these patients are often pleased by an increase in physician empathy and a reduction in the power imbalance between the doctor and themselves. On the other hand, some physicians have poignantly described (see Suggested Readings) the emotional and social withdrawal of their colleagues when they have become ill or developed a disability.

There are other practical concerns related to the impact of an illness on the practice, including income loss, ability to continue practicing, practice or call coverage, insurability, and, at times, remaining licensed or credentialed.

The final set of concerns has to do with the reaction of the physician's family or loved ones. Some physicians have family relationships characterized by power inequities, and the vulnerability of an illness may create a fear of losing power or control. The physician may be fearful of testing how supportive family members can be in a crisis. This may reflect an unrealistic fear of being disappointed, or it may be a realistic appraisal of a family that has simply grown less connected over time or has withdrawn from the physician as a result of neglect, abuse, or estrangement. In either case, the fear of facing an illness without adequate social support may be especially daunting.

The Assessment

Even after they decide that some evaluation is necessary, many physicians will follow a circuitous path.

> **Case Vignette.** Dr S, a 26-year-old intern, slipped on the ice and fell with his wrist extended as he was rushing to begin an emergency department shift. Because of the pain, he had an x-ray taken almost immediately, and it revealed no fracture. He continued to work with a great deal of pain for the next week until his chief resident noticed his difficulties performing all procedures. When the chief resident heard the story, he ordered Dr S to see an orthopedic surgeon, who immediately casted him to protect against a possible navicular bone fracture, something that should have been done right after the injury.

Rather than seek out their personal physician (even if they have one), some physicians will instead undertake a process of self-diagnosis. This is more likely if any testing can be done without involving a colleague, such as ordering blood tests, and these may even be submitted under a patient's or family member's name. Tests that require another physician's execution or interpretation, such as radiologic studies, may be avoided. Sometimes assessment is bypassed in favor of empiric self-treatment trials, generally from office samples or self-prescribed. Particularly in the case of using anxiolytics or opiate analgesics, this can lead to additional clinical problems (substance abuse) or legal problems (in some states, self-prescribing of controlled substances is illegal).

Physicians may try to get assistance from a colleague via a "curbside consultation," and this may even be done without disclosing that the physician is the one with the symptoms, pretending instead that it is a patient in one's own practice. There may be special reluctance to seek out a colleague directly if the physician suspects an illness that is stigmatized (HIV or other sexual transmitted diseases, substance abuse, depression, etc).

Even when a colleague is consulted, there may be further twists. Bynder noted that physicians often selected a physician on the basis of social or professional relationships rather than solely on the basis of expertise. At times the process of self-diagnosis may have advanced to the stage where an inappropriate specialist is selected because of an erroneous presumption about the cause of a symptom (eg, consulting a neurologist for dizziness with a vascular, otologic, or anxiety disorder cause). And even if an appropriate colleague is consulted, the history may be intentionally or inadvertently presented in such a way as to deter or elicit certain diagnoses or treatment recommendations.

Coping with Illness

As noted earlier, there are as many adaptations to an illness as there are patients, even when the patient is a physician. Because many physicians have certain typical personality traits and have adopted certain medical values, some reactions to illness are perhaps more characteristic among physicians than in the general population. Even after a diagnosis is reached and an initial treatment plan developed, many of the factors that may have delayed or complicated reaching a diagnosis may reemerge to affect the adaptation phase. There may be a resumption of minimization and nondisclosure of new symptoms or of self-diagnosing, self-test ordering, and self-prescribing, usually rationalized as "not wanting to trouble [my] colleague who is treating me." This, of course, can lead to fragmentation and poor coordination of care, not to mention the risk of self-malpractice.

Control Issues. As noted in Chapter 2, physicians as a rule tend to be quite preoccupied with maintenance of control over themselves, others, their feelings, and, where possible, the future. Almost any illness can have devastating effects on one's ability to control things. Table 12-2 shows a partial list of some of the things that can be wrested from physician-patients' control. As much as the physician would like to script the symptom picture, illness course, and prognosis, this quickly becomes impossible with almost all conditions. Similarly, the emotional reactions engendered by the illness or its effects can leave the physician feeling that his or her emotions, generally under tight control when healthy, are now running wild. And the interpersonal and emotional reactions of those around the physician follow their own course rather than being more rigidly defined by established roles and their scripts.

Table 12-2
Elements of How an Illness Can Diminish Control

☐ Ability to function in expected roles
☐ Change in bodily functions
☐ Level of physical comfort
☐ Need for assistance from others
☐ Presence or absence of a symptom
☐ Course of the illness
☐ Prognosis of the illness
☐ Emotions in reaction to the illness
☐ Reactions of others to one's condition
☐ Financial impact

Obsessionalism. Many doctors normally feel that they are in a constant struggle to know enough and to be sufficiently certain in their decision making. This trait can be vastly amplified when the decisions to be made may affect their lives and careers. One way that physicians may deal with the ambiguities inherent in an illness is by researching the factual information about it. This at times can be quite adaptive, but in some cases it is done compulsively, leading to no resolution of any ambiguities and risking alienation of caregivers (by second-guessing, pestering for information, or exhibiting one-upsmanship maneuvers). An opposite but less common reaction is for the physician-patient to become very passive, turn all information gathering and decision making over to the treating physician, and in effect allow the treater to be the bearer of the uncertainties.

Omnipotence and Role Definition. Some physicians are extremely concerned about appearing weak or vulnerable, and they tend to hide these anxieties with shows of overconfidence and bravado. Along similar lines, they are often reluctant to ask for help because they fear it will not be forthcoming or will come with an unacceptable price tag attached. These phenomena in an ailing physician may lead to avoidance of sufficient care, over-estimation of functional abilities, or reluctance to acknowledge distress. Many physicians have built so much of their professional and personal lives around the one role of "doctor" that it can be very difficult for them to adopt other social roles even when appropriate. One reason that even a not overly serious illness can sometimes be so devastating to physicians is because of their difficulty reaching out for and accepting help and support. This is because of their often limited ability to act as a friend, partner, or parent or in another social role when they are temporarily robbed of the physician's mantle.

The Physician as Patient and the Health Care System

Much of the health care system is highly physician centered, so it too struggles when the patient is a physician. There is a strong tendency on the part of treating physicians and other health professionals to allow the physician-patient to keep his/her role as much as possible, both out of habit and because of a sense of identification with the patient's plight. When this works well, it may allow the physician-patient to experience less vulnerability and narcissistic injury than would otherwise be the case. On the other hand, it can also lead to compromised care.

> **Case Vignette**. Dr C, a radiologist, consulted Dr J, his internist, about several brief episodes of left-sided weakness that he had experienced in the previous few months. Dr J, after a careful evaluation, told Dr C that these were almost certainly transient ischemic attacks and recommended that Dr C "take a little aspirin." Because he assumed that Dr C knew all about such things, Dr J did not go over the actual risk of future stroke, nor did he discuss any possible changes in Dr C's diet, exercise, or hypertension or lipid-lowering regimens. Dr C began to feel that he was "doomed," because he greatly overestimated his risk of stroke, and he interpreted the lack

of discussion about risk factors as evidence that there was nothing he could do to affect his risk. He began taking four aspirin tablets a day, an amount he considered "little" because it was far less than he had taken years earlier for an arthritic condition.

There is often a strong tendency on the part of health care providers to believe that physician-patients will be knowledgeable about their illnesses and treatments, so imparting of information may be cursory when compared to what is offered nonphysician patients. This is part of what has been referred to as the "VIP syndrome," where certain "special" patients have the usual medical care rules stretched or are exempted entirely from following them. Besides patient education lapses, this can include cursory histories and abbreviated physical exams "to avoid embarrassment" (and thus missing the alcoholism, rectal mass, or increased anesthesia risk); skipping "unpleasant" steps in testing (eg, inadequate bowel prep leading to repeated x-rays or colonoscopy); overutilizing testing or consultants; being less aggressive than usual in interventions (to reduce the risk of adverse outcomes); or neglecting reporting or other requirements (eg, failing to report a sexually transmitted disease to public health authorities or seizures to the state drivers' license office).

Because the treating physician and the physician-patient are often colleagues, the doctor-patient relationship may be at risk for boundary transgressions (see Chapter 9). The treating physician may overidentify with the patient, and he/she may therefore offer advice based on his or her personal values rather than the patient's. There may be issues about when (before or after hours when no one else is around?) and where (office? patient's home? doctor's lounge?) to see the patient, confidentiality, and fees that can become thorny when colleagues are treated.

Other health care professionals may experience difficulties with physician-patients when they are treated as VIPs. Office staff may be unhappy with disruptions in office functioning, technicians may resent off-hours testing, and hospital nurses may be unhappy about ward routines not being followed. Tensions may be compounded if the patient or family acts with a sense of entitlement rather than appreciation. There may also be awkwardness that comes from seeing a staff physician in a setting and role different from usual.

Reactions of Those Around the Physician-patient

An illness never affects the patient alone: the patient's support system, his/her caregivers, and others are all pulled into the process, by choice or by circumstance.

> **Case Vignette.** Dr Y, a psychiatrist, had been treating Ms M for many years. Despite his experience and skill, she remained very mistrustful and aloof, and he constantly felt that she was reluctant to tell him much of what troubled her. He saw her late one afternoon at the end of a long day of sitting with patients, and after she left he decided to attend to his hemorrhoids, which had been getting more painful as the day wore on. Just as he was crouched over and inserting a rectal suppository, Ms M returned unexpectedly to recover the gloves that she had forgotten in Dr Y's office. Dr Y was mortified, but the patient grinned from ear to ear at the sight, and she announced, "Well, maybe you are a human being and not a deity after all." She left, and from that point forward Dr Y found that she was far more forthcoming in sharing her problems.

Families/Support Networks

There are as many family reactions as there are families and physicians. Table 12-3 lists some of the factors that need to be considered when trying to understand the impact of an illness on a family (see Rolland for a thorough description). All family members bring to the situation their personal and familial experiences with illness, their own understanding of the meaning of the illness,* their relationship with the patient, and their alliances and conflicts with other family members.

Some physicians' families are characterized by strained relationships with the physician because of interpersonal distance caused by work

---

* This is the "cultural interpretation" of the illness, which includes its cause, its cure, its significance (eg, whether it is a sign or punishment), and so on.

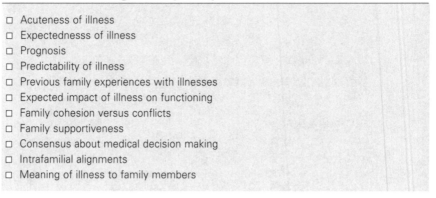

Table 12-3
Factors Affecting Family Response to Illness

- ☐ Acuteness of illness
- ☐ Expectednesss of illness
- ☐ Prognosis
- ☐ Predictability of illness
- ☐ Previous family experiences with illnesses
- ☐ Expected impact of illness on functioning
- ☐ Family cohesion versus conflicts
- ☐ Family supportiveness
- ☐ Consensus about medical decision making
- ☐ Intrafamilial alignments
- ☐ Meaning of illness to family members

demands, emotional detachment, or both. This may be particularly an issue when both members of an intimate partnership are physicians. The pull of an illness can at times draw a family together as the interpersonal contacts increase and deepen, but at times the bonds will have atrophied or the resentments grown too great over the years. Physicians craving closeness and support on account of illness may find that family members are unwilling to rally in support of someone whom they had not found to be supportive earlier when he/she was well. There may also be unspoken beliefs that certain illnesses (eg, myocardial infarction) are just deserts for the physician's having adopted a high-stress lifestyle.

Patients

Doctors almost universally fear that if patients are made aware of the doctor's illness or limitations, it would result in a loss of trust and face. This may well be the case with certain socially stigmatized conditions, at least for most patients (although doctors recovering from substance use disorders frequently describe the encouragement they receive from their patients dealing with their own addictions). However, the inevitable power imbalance between doctor and patient is generally much more appreciated by the doctor, so that when the physician's illness evens the balance somewhat, patients are frequently quite pleased. Although they express their sympathy, many also describe their relief at seeing the doctor as more of an equal. They also believe that the doctor who has been ill will be more empathic with regard to their suffering, and in fact many doctors who have been sick do describe an increased appreciation for what their patients experience. Only rarely do patients express an unwillingness to work with a physician they had known and liked who has a new disability, and this can often be overcome when the physician demonstrates that his/her competence remains intact.

Colleagues

The reaction of physicians to a colleague's illness is highly variable. If the relationship had been a friendly one before the illness, there is often a showing of support, whether practical (coverage, loans, etc) or emotional. Unfortunately, many physicians regard the state of being ill as a possibly contagious one and avoid contact with suffering colleagues. This is thought to have to do with often unconscious exaggerated fears of sickness and death and the magical thinking of believing that a sick physician too openly shows the limitations of medicine and physicians.

Other Health Care Professionals

The reactions of nonphysician health care workers who collaborate with a physician to a physician's illness are variable. In general, other health professionals are probably less uncomfortable with illness than are physicians, and they may be far more willing to be supportive and demonstrative. On the other hand, if physicians have engendered ill will with these professionals in the manner described above for physician families, such collegial support may be less forthcoming.

Summary

In general, physicians experience difficulties accepting the sick role, and so their willingness to seek care and be treated as are other patients is diminished. This reluctance can lead to poorer medical outcomes for the physician-patient and to more interpersonal difficulties with health care professionals. The assistance provided by the physician's social support network is largely a function of the degree to which the individual relationships with family, colleagues, and others have been properly maintained in the past. Caregivers and family members can be helpful by being sensitive to the extra vulnerabilities already existing in the physician struggling with an illness.

Suggested Readings

Alliborne A, Oakes D, Shannon HS. The health and healthcare of doctors. *J R Coll Gen Prac.* 1981;31:728-734.

Aoun H. From the eye of the storm, with the eyes of a physician. *Ann Intern Med.* 1992;116:335-338.

Bynder H. Doctors as patients: a study of the medical care of physicians and their families. *Med Care.* 1968;6:157-167.

La Puma J, Stocking C, La Voie D, et al. When physicians treat members of their own families: practices in a community hospital. *N Engl J Med.* 1991;325:1290-1294.

Mandell H, Spiro M, eds. *When Doctors Get Sick.* New York: Plenum Medical; 1987.

Marzuk PM. When the patient is a physician. *N Engl J Med.* 1987;317:1409-1411.

Rabin D, Rabin PL, Rabin R. Compounding the ordeal of ALS: isolation from my fellow physicians. *N Engl J Med.* 1982;307:506-509.

Robbins GT, MacDonald MC, Pack GT. Delays in the diagnosis and treatment of physicians with cancer. *Cancer.* 1953;6:624-626.

Rolland JS. *Families, Illness, and Disability: An Integrative Treatment Model.* New York: Basic Books; 1994.

Rosenbaum EE. *A Taste of My Own Medicine: When the Doctor Is the Patient.* New York: Random House; 1988.

Schneck SA. "Doctoring" doctors and their families. *JAMA.* 1998;280:2039-2042.

Stetten D. Coping with blindness. *N Engl J Med.* 1981;305:458-460.

Stoudemire A, Rhoads JM. When the doctor needs a doctor: special considerations for the physician-patient. *Ann Intern Med.* 1983;98:654-659.

Weintraub W. "The VIP syndrome": a clinical study in hospital psychiatry. *J Nerv Ment Dis.* 1964;138:181-193.

Chapter 13

Troubled or Troubling Physicians: Administrative Responses

George J. Van Komen, MD

D octors too become ill. The healer sometimes desperately needs to be healed. Physicians when afflicted with illness must be afforded the same care, the same concern, and the same attention as that provided to all patients. But a physician's illness, when compared to that of a standard patient, is more complicated, much more difficult because of the doctor's direct association with the medical profession. A physician's emotional response to an illness is also much different. Doctors have a real, well-founded concern that shunning will occur not only from patients but also from colleagues. Enormous guilt will frequently accompany a physician's illness, further complicating the patient-doctor from coming forward to medical associates for help and needed treatment.

A number of organizations, both private and governmental, as they become aware of a doctor's illness, may also become concerned and interact. These organizations may include state and local medical societies, hospitals where the doctor has medical staff privileges, and the state's physician licensing board through which the doctor obtained a medical license.

Because of these many complicating aspects of a physician's illnesses, especially when his/her illness involves regulatory committees and boards, the physician perceives that there is a real potential for great loss, not only in the form of patients but also in potential future earnings. When physicians are sick, they will dwell endlessly on how patients, colleagues, and others will view their illness. If the illness is perceived as being psychological or mental, heightened caution will often further delay appropriate medical intervention and treatment.

The purpose of this chapter will be to explore some of the medical maladies, psychological illnesses, and behavioral problems physicians acquire or display and show how these disorders may impact their relationships with hospital medical staffs, credentialing and privileging bodies, and state medical licensing agencies or boards. Also carefully examined will be common feelings and actions taken by doctors when they perceive that their health problems may impact their medical practices, their income, hospital privileges, and medical licensing.

Physicians develop all the physical, mental, emotional, and behavioral problems seen in other patients. These medical problems include health problems such as the aging process, dementia, the physical and metabolic problems of a medical disorder, and mental problems, which include drug and alcohol abuse, depression, manic-depression, anxiety syndromes, thought disorders, and a myriad of behavioral problems. Behavioral problems may fall into categories such as boundary crossing with sexual abuse of patients and forms of disruptive and problematic behavior. Nearly 75% of physicians who come before their state medical boards are there because of problems involving the abuse of alcohol or other drugs.

Regulatory Groups

Many organizations and groups are charged with the duty to improve the quality of health care that is provided in our country. They do this by regularly evaluating physician skills. State licensing bodies have the specific responsibility to protect the public from harm that can come from improperly trained and skilled physicians. Hospitals and other health care organizations likewise are concerned and have a responsibility to their patients that the medical care they receive is appropriate and of high caliber. State and local medical societies help physicians deal with the many challenges facing doctors, including the challenge to help physicians deliver medical care at a high standard.

State Physician Licensing Boards

State physician licensing boards are composed of physicians, public members, and, occasionally, other health care providers. The primary responsibility and obligation of every state licensing body is to protect consumers of health care through proper licensing and the regulation of physicians practicing within their state.

Physicians must know and accept that the practice of medicine is not an inherent right of an individual, but a privilege granted by the people of their state to physicians through their elected representatives. To protect the public from the unprofessional, improper, and incompetent practice of medicine, it is necessary for the state to provide laws and regulations that outline the practice of medicine. The primary role of each licensing board is therefore to regulate the practice of medicine in their respective state. The guidance for this regulation is outlined in state statues and is usually called the *Medical Practice Act.*

Through the process of licensure, each state ensures that practicing physicians have appropriate education and training, and that physicians abide by recognized standards of professional conduct while serving their patients. Candidates for licensure must also pass rigorous examinations, which were designed to assess a physician's ability to apply knowledge, concepts, and principles that are important in health and disease. This combined knowledge constitutes the basis for physicians to deliver safe and effective patient care.

Another responsibility with which each licensing board is charged is to evaluate whether a physician's professional conduct warrants modification of his/her medical license. The information used to evaluate a physician's professional conduct is received from consumer complaints, malpractice data, information from physicians, hospitals, and other health-care institutions, and reports from other government agencies.

Often the complaints received involve a physician's health, such as a problem with drug or alcohol abuse or another mental illness. Licensing boards are always sensitive to a physician's health and are interested in securing appropriate health care for an ill physician, but the board must also follow its other responsibility to protect the public to whom the doctor is providing health care.

When a complaint about a physician is received, that complaint is carefully evaluated. When the health of a physician is involved, appropriate referral and contacts are made to ensure that the physician receives proper health care. Physicians on licensing boards are concerned about physician well-being, and an important part of their commitment to their colleagues is to see them receive proper and appropriate medical care. But if there is substantial reason to believe that the physician has violated the law, an investigation will be conducted, which may result in a hearing or other discipline being imposed.

Examples of unprofessional conduct by a physician that come to licensing board attention include the following:

- physical or sexual abuse of a patient
- prescribing drugs in excessive amounts or without legitimate reason
- impaired ability to practice because of addiction, or physical or mental illness
- dishonesty
- conviction of a felony
- delegating the practice of medicine to an unlicensed individual
- not recognizing or acting on common symptoms
- failing to meet continuing medical education requirements

Many of these failings are the result of behavioral problems rather than general medical or mental illnesses. It is also important to note that minor disagreements do not fall under unprofessional conduct, nor does poor "customer service."

Due process is afforded to any physician who has a complaint brought against him/her. Due process states that an individual is innocent until proven guilty. Each physician is assured that he or she will be treated fairly, not arbitrarily, and very reasonably. In the rare instance of severe egregious behavior by a physician, the medical board does have the authority to summarily suspend a physician's license until an administrative hearing before a judge can be scheduled and conducted.

A medical board never focuses on punishing physicians, but rather on protecting the public and helping physicians who have physical and mental health problems, as well as behavioral or ethical problems. Medical help will almost always be recommended for physicians who have medical problems, either physical or mental, that have interfered with their overall ability to practice high-quality and appropriate medicine. However, a physician must realize that for serious ethical or behavioral problems and other egregious violations, restrictions, probation, or other sanctions may need to be imposed on their license. In cases where medical help will benefit the physician, this will be recommended. Through this way, both the public will be protected and the valuable asset to society of the physician practicing medicine will be maintained. All physicians who practice medicine must realize and accept that the improvement of the health and circumstance of patients is the primary goal within the medical profession.

With the privilege to practice medicine in the United States come important responsibilities in regard to controlled substances, both prescription medications and illegal controlled drugs. Because of the high prevalence of addictive disease in our society, each physician should have an understanding of the process of addiction. This will not only help the doctor to appropriately and properly prescribe and use controlled substances, but also help the physician to recognize addictive behavior in associates and also protect against self-abuse, the medical problem, as previously mentioned, that most frequently brings physicians before state licensing boards.

Physician Diversion Programs

Laws have been established throughout the United States allowing physicians to seek treatment and medical care for their chemical dependency without having to face disciplinary action. If a physician has a chemical dependency problem and meets certain requirements, a referral by the state medical board and administrative staff may be made to a state-run "diversion" program. This program allows the physician to be treated and receive aftercare without formal discipline by the state medical board and without the painful sting of public disclosure. In diversion programs, physicians may receive counseling and treatment, be monitored as to progress, participate in support groups, and have their practices observed, all within the confidentiality of the diversion program.

Certain requirements, however, must be met by participating physicians in diversion programs as opposed to appearing before state medical boards. The purpose of diversion programs is not only to rehabilitate the physician, but also to carefully protect the safety of the public. For example, certain physician behaviors, such as having diverted drugs to patients or others, may disqualify a doctor from participating in a diversion program, primarily because this type of action puts not only the physician but the public at risk. Diversion programs will only work when the total safety of the public is ensured. At the onset of a physician's participation in a diversion program, an agreement is made that if, during the treatment period, the physician is determined to be unable to work safely, he or she must be willing to give up practicing medicine during the time it is deemed unsafe. When the physician does return to practice there may be monitoring and certain levels of practice restrictions. Experience with diversion programs has shown that physician rehabilitation can be accomplished in total confidence and still allow the public to be protected. Successful diversion programs have now shown that physicians do not need to be publicly disgraced through an adversarial formal discipline process to be successfully returned to full-time duty and remain a valuable asset to society.

Illnesses and Impairment

Physician impairment is defined as the inability to practice medicine with reasonable skill and safety because of physical or mental illness. Some of the causes of impairment include alcohol and other chemical drug dependencies and mood disorders, which may adversely affect a physician's decision-making capabilities, medical judgment, and competence. Other mental illnesses that can render a physician impaired to practice medicine include severe panic disorder, obsessive-compulsive disorder, posttraumatic stress disorders, eating disorders, and certain forms of adjustment and personality disorders.

Organic impairment problems may also affect a physician. Aging-related complications may significantly impair a physician's cognition, memory, and ability to safely fulfill responsibilities. Cognitive and memory impairment may also develop after drug or alcohol addiction, after a drug overdose, or from poisoning by toxins such as carbon monoxide. Delirious states may result from metabolic impairments from a wide range of medical illness. A dementia may develop in association with neurologic conditions such as Alzheimer's disease, vascular disorders, Parkinson's disease, head trauma, multiple sclerosis, and AIDS. When mental capacity impairment is suspected, a careful psychiatric assessment and mental status examination must be conducted to assure the public that the physician's skills and capabilities have not been impaired to a point that the physician's patients would be put at risk.

Reports as to the frequency of physician impairment in the United States range from 7% to 10%. Of all the impairments, the most common impairments are those caused by dependence on alcohol or other chemical substances. Many of the physicians who have a chemical dependence also suffer from a comorbid psychiatric disorder (dual diagnosis). These physicians may also have a major depression, bipolar illness, panic disorder, obsessive-compulsive disorder, or other significant psychiatric illnesses. These dual diagnostic disorders are more difficult to treat because of the addictive disorder, and will therefore require intensive proper treatment. For appropriate care to be rendered, a harmonious and trusting cooperation must be present among the physician-patient, the medical team rendering the care, hospital committees concerned about the physician's health, and the state regulatory bodies. Only through this type of mutual collaboration will recovery be possible.

Prejudices from those within the medical profession toward physicians who seek help or care for their mental illnesses must never occur. This is essential for physicians to seek help. Unrecognized and untreated physician impairment is both egregious and heartbreaking in its potential for harm. Physicians should be able to speak openly about their illnesses without being stigmatized or viewed negatively by those within the physician community.

A special word is in order about HIV/AIDS. An HIV-infected physician must be treated with compassion and due respect to rights, privacy, and the strictest confidentiality. A physician with HIV does have the professional obligation to "do no harm," in terms of both transmission of the illness and the presence of any neuropsychiatric impairment. State licensing boards in cooperation with HIV-infected physicians must design a practice plan that will protect the public while still allowing the afflicted physician avenues to practice with appropriate modifications to protect all patients from any potential harm. Restrictions of any sort based solely on the HIV infection itself are wholly unwarranted and discriminatory.

Addictive Diseases

To recognize the addictive process is not necessarily difficult. Addiction has been characterized as an unmanageable life filled with dishonesty. The process of addiction is complex, often lifelong, and frequently familial. An addict is an individual who uses drugs, such as prescription controlled substances or illicit street drugs, in a nontherapeutic way to make himself or herself feel good. They frequently, however, do this in a most self-destructive way. Physicians rapidly come to recognize that addicts who are in their practice behave and act demonstratively in a deleterious way, not at all in their own self-interest. The clinical aspects of this topic are covered more fully in Chapter 8.

There are four characteristics present in every addict. These four features are to addiction as cough or fever are to pneumonia. These four descriptive features of each patient with addiction are as follows:

1. *Loss of control.* Addiction is a compulsive disorder. Addicts have lost their ability to regulate the use of alcohol or other drugs. They have crossed an invisible line. Once they have crossed this line they will forever have difficulty in maintaining control. To lose control feels bad. Addicts make up their mind each day not to use drugs, but during each day they lose control and they use. Losing control, whether with drugs or with any other behavior, makes an individual feel terrible.

2. *Continued use despite adverse consequences.* As mentioned, each addict attempts to stay in control, but no matter how serious the attempt, an addict will continually, time and time again, lose control. By definition, addiction is a disease that continues despite punishment for this loss of control. Addicts are always in trouble, with their family, other acquaintances, or the law. Incarceration, by definition, will not cure the truly established addict. Adverse health consequences by addicted patients are nearly always neglected. Addicts know that if they continue to use, their addiction may kill them, but the addictive disease compels them to continue despite these potential adverse consequences.

3. *Craving.* The daily symptom of addiction is craving. This incredible craving is the intense preoccupation to get and use a drug. Another term interchangeably used for craving is *drug hunger.* Neurophysiologists tell us that craving comes from the same brain center from which thirst and hunger originate. Knowing this, one can appreciate how uncomfortable a drug addict must feel when he or she experiences the same unpleasant craving as we would feel if food or drink were to be withheld from us for a prolonged period of time, such as for several days.

4. *Denial.* This is the most misunderstood feature of addiction. Denial is the willingness of an addict to take risks to obtain the drug he or she craves despite the overwhelming odds that he or she will be caught and punished. An addict is in true denial when, under the intense pressure of craving to use a drug, he or she does not see the adverse consequences associated with his or her continued use.

Fortunately, much progress has been made during the past years not only with the identification of physicians who have become impaired from substance abuse, but also in their treatment. Aggressive intervention and treatment programs have become commonplace. Hospital medical and administrative staffs, medical societies, and state medical boards have regularly joined together to assist in the treatment and rehabilitation of impaired physicians. Many state legislatures have passed laws allowing physicians to participate in physician diversion programs. These programs allow physicians to receive adequate treatment and follow-up care in anonymity, allowing physicians to maintain their position and respect with patients within their communities. Early recognition of the addictive disease process is the key element that allows medical boards and other organizations to institute therapy rather than taking punitive actions.

Depression

By the very nature of the high frequency of depression in the public at large, depression is also very common among physicians. Studies have shown that physicians develop clinical depression at rates comparable to those in the general public, but a physician's response to depression is frequently quite different. Although physicians often sense the diagnosis of depression, they delay treatment and intervention because of fears as to how their families, their colleagues and the established medical regulatory system will respond. A physician may self-administer antidepressant medications in the hope of preventing the guilt and embarrassment they feel when they are depressed. Having an understanding of the disease process, depressed physicians may choose to withdraw in an attempt to conceal their depression from peers and medical associates, an unfortunate decision that is usually counterproductive for the recovery and stabilization of the disease.

If physicians are to receive early and adequate treatment for depression and mental illnesses, they must look at these diseases in themselves and colleagues in a different light from what is done presently. Doctors must learn to help and support each other. Afflicted physicians should become more comfortable in sharing their medical or psychological problems in confidence with other physicians.

Fortunately, there are some physicians who are beginning to speak out and discuss more openly their health and psychological problems. Recently, the president of the Utah Medical Association shared his feelings and his struggle with depression in his monthly President's Message in the *Utah Medical Bulletin*. His remarkable and landmark article is shared with his permission in this chapter's Appendix.

This new, commendable openness of this outstanding leader in medicine about his own depression, as well as that of other physicians, will pave the way for doctors to change their attitudes not only toward the mental disease of depression but also toward all mental and psychological disorders that may occur in physician colleagues. Most importantly, however, openness such as this article contains will help doctors realize that, even as a physician, having an illness is normal and is all right. Through more openness, physicians will come to realize that treatment for mental diseases is available and that sympathetic physician colleagues will be there to help.

Physician Misconduct

Misprescribing of Controlled Substances

Many newspaper headlines have chronicled improper prescribing of controlled drugs by physicians. Failure to safeguard medical practices through inappropriate prescribing may result in serious discipline from state medical boards. These problems almost always could have been avoided through pertinent education and by setting appropriate practice guidelines.

Each year thousands of physicians throughout the United States are disciplined because of drug- related problems. The misuse of controlled substances by physicians can be devastating to the ability of doctors to practice medicine and to the well-being and health of patients and to themselves. The American Medical Association, in an effort to assist and aid physicians in understanding drug-related problems encountered in medical practices, has classified physician misprescribing in four categories. They are referred to as the "four D's" of misprescribing: dishonest, disabled, dated, and deceived.

1. *Dishonest* physicians are a "black eye" to our profession. These practitioners have learned that profits are high in prescription-writing fraud. They are not concerned about their "patient's" health.

2. *Disabled* physicians have themselves become addicted to drugs or alcohol. They frequently devise creative schemes to obtain controlled drugs for their own addictive cravings. Their judgment has been distorted by their addiction, leading them to overprescribe to their patients.

3. *Dated* physicians are those who do not keep current with advances in medicine. They are often busy, overworked, and conscientious doctors who believe their patients need them so much that they cannot take time off for postgraduate study. They continue to use dangerous drugs to treat particular ailments even though newer, safer therapy is available.

4. *Deceived* physicians are mostly caring and trusting physicians. In their enthusiasm to help everyone, however, they become victims of the deceptive plots of drug addicts, who seek prescription drugs either to fuel their own habits or for resale on the streets. These physicians often have only a rudimentary knowledge of the drug addictive process.

Physicians can develop a safe and appropriate prescribing practice. There are a number of safeguards that every physician must understand. These principles must be learned and applied to daily practice. An important element is to understand drug addiction, and then to apply good medical evaluation whenever a controlled substance prescription is used. Physicians can have a rewarding practice, devoid of concerns of actions from regulatory bodies, if they understand their responsibility to keep the misuse, abuse, and potential diversion of controlled drugs as low as possible. Physicians who misprescribe may be referred by their licensing board to one of several programs that serve to educate them about optimal controlled drug prescribing practices (see Chapter 15).

Sexual Misconduct

One of the major behavior problems occurring within physician practices is the unfortunate crossing of boundaries. This frequently results in sexual improprieties and sexual violations. Physicians must understand that sexual misconduct is not related to either a mental or a physical illness, but rather is a serious lapse in the ethical conduct and behavior of a doctor. A physician should understand the difference between a sexual boundary crossing in the course of medical practice and a psychological or medical health problem. While *sexual addiction* is a frequently used phrase, this condition is not recognized as a disease in the American Psychiatric Association's *Diagnostic and Statistical Manual of Mental Disorders, Fourth Edition* (DSM-IV). While a mental disorder may be the claim for the cause of sexual misconduct, physicians must understand that state medical boards do not recognize that sexual misconduct is caused by a physical or mental illness.

Sexual misconduct is defined as an intolerable violation of the public's trust. This type of physician behavior will never be acceptable or tolerated either by the general public or by the medical profession. Yet, despite strong sanctions against physician sexual misconduct, newspaper headlines continue to blare out across our country about sexual violations committed by physicians. Sensational headlines such as "Physician Denies Fondling Patients," "Doctor Molested Me, Woman Says," "Local Surgeon Accused of Sexual Misconduct on Job," "Doctor Gives Up License Amid More Sex Allegations," and "MD Found Guilty of Sexual Impropriety" cover the front pages of our country's newspapers.

There is nothing more tragic than when physicians cross these established boundaries and entangle their personal sexual desires with their medical practices. Doctors stand to lose not only their medical licenses but also their reputations in their practicing communities. Physicians must recognize that inappropriate sexual boundary crossing may cause patients deep emotional suffering and often irreversible psychological and physical trauma.

Physicians must be aware of the increasing number of complaints throughout our country regarding sexual misconduct. A practicing doctor must understand what constitutes sexual misconduct in a medical practice. Because of an imbalance of power, there has been a traditional ban since the time of Hippocrates on the sexual exploitation of the physician-patient relationship. Through education, physicians can come to understand and recognize acceptable behavior in regard to sexual boundary issues. With this knowledge, physicians can protect their practices from violations of these important boundaries and also reduce potential patient harm.

Physician sexual misconduct is defined as behavior that exploits the physician-patient relationship in a sexual way. There are two levels of severity of sexual misconduct. The two categories of sexual misconduct are sexual violations and sexual improprieties. Although sexual violations are considered to be more serious than sexual improprieties, both categories may be the basis for harsh disciplinary actions by state medical boards. Sexual violations include any form of physician-patient sex, whether it is initiated by the doctor or the patient. In a physician-patient relationship, these is no such thing as "consensual sex." Sexual violations may include, but are not limited to, the touching of breasts, genitals, or any sexualized body part for any purpose other than appropriate examination or treatment. Kissing a patient in a romantic or sexual way may be considered a sexual violation. Sexual improprieties, however, usually encompass behaviors, gestures, or expressions that are seductive, sexually suggestive, or sexually demeaning to a patient. Examples of sexual improprieties may include, among others, deliberately watching a patient dress or undress, making sexual comments about a patient's body or underclothing, making comments about potential sexual performance during an examination except when the examination is pertinent to the issue of sexual function or dysfunction, or the making of sexualized or sexually demeaning comments to a patient.

Clear and concise professional standards established by the American Medical Association (AMA) should help physicians avoid any sexual misconduct problems. The AMA Council of Ethical and Judicial Affairs has set as basics the following four standards:

1. Sexual contact or a romantic relationship concurrent with the physician-patient relationship is unethical.

2. Sexual contact with a former patient, under certain circumstances, may be unethical.

3. Physicians should be educated about the extremely important ethical issues involved with sexual misconduct.

4. When a medical colleague commits sexual misconduct, reporting is important and ethically appropriate. In fact, if physicians decide not to report a colleague, they may be in violation of their own ethical responsibilities.

Having a "consensual" sexual relationship with a patient under any circumstance is not acceptable. In fact, even the termination of the physician-patient relationship does not eliminate the possibility that sexual contact between a physician and a former patient may still be unethical. Many physicians who are charged with sexual misconduct blame the patient for the unprofessional sexual relationships. A physician must recognize that, even if the patient is unusually seductive, it is *never* the patient's fault or responsibility. The physician is the individual who has the ethical guidelines and must act accordingly, regardless of what the patient does. The physician-patient relationship is based on trust, and the physician is clearly always the trustee.

Experts who deal with physician sexual misconduct have identified certain characteristics of physicians who are at risk. Some of the characteristics of at-risk physicians include undue physical touch, making sensual comments to patients, and the discussing of their own personal matters with their patients, such as their marriages or their own sexual or family problems. Other risky features include unusual practices, such as late hours without staff, making unnecessary house calls, and practicing while impaired from alcohol or other drugs. See Chapter 9 for more information about those who perpetrate this type of misconduct.

Many serious consequences may follow for physicians who engage in sexual misconduct. State licensing agencies, ethics committees of professional organizations, malpractice litigation, and civil and criminal statutes all have the potential to impose sanctions, which may be very harsh. "A $40 night in a motel room can quickly become a $1 million lawsuit," reads a recent position statement from the Federation of State Medical Boards. An inappropriate sexual act has the potential to interrupt a hard-won medical career, one that may never be reestablished. An appropriate and honest question for every physician should be, "What can I do to protect myself from being charged with sexual misconduct?" Every physician must recognize that he or she under certain circumstances may be vulnerable. Personal problems, such as divorce, separation, loss of a child or spouse, or other times of personal stress may predispose physicians to breach their value systems.

Denial and defensiveness are prominent responses by doctors who have engaged in sexual misconduct. "I did it because I have a bad marriage" and "It was her fault, she came on to me" are two customary responses from physicians. Studies have shown that it is unusual for professional sexual misconduct to include only one patient. The more common experience is one of predatory behavior wherein multiple patients have been violated.

Physicians must recognize that sexual misconduct usually begins with relatively minor boundary violations. Physicians can avoid going down the "slippery slope" to sexual misconduct by adhering to the following suggestions.

1. *Do not seek emotional support from patients.* Discussions with patients regarding personal marital problems or sexual fantasies is altogether inappropriate.

2. *Do not ask patients to perform personal services for you.* Giving patients rides home from the office in your car, or having contact during social events, gives the impression that the patient-physician relationship may have been breached. Keep relationships as professional as possible.

3. *Never do an intimate examination on a patient of the opposite sex without a chaperone.* Patients should be seen and examined, as much as possible, in the office with a chaperone, where appropriate.

4. *Recognize your own vulnerability*. Be acquainted with the profile or characteristics of patients who are predisposed to becoming involved in professional sexual misconduct.

5. *Be careful when exchanging gifts with patients*. Also avoid giving certain patients special billing advantages or fees. Within the investigation of sexual boundary violations, fact finders or investigators may question what type of currency was paid, and what sort of special discounts or privileges were afforded to the patient.

6. *Exchanging hugs with patients may be allowed cautiously, within an appropriate context or situation*. This may be perceived as a finicky suggestion, but being cautious in these types of situations is prudent. If hugs are to be shared, make certain that the patient grants consent, and having another person present is certainly advisable.

7. *Give an appropriate response and warning if a patient is aggressively seductive*. A firm but kindly given response can save both patient and physician much heartache. A suggested physician response may be as follows: "This behavior is inappropriate and is not in the best interest of our professional relationship."

A physician-patient relationship is built upon confidence and trust. The physician is always the one who sets these standards and makes certain that they are maintained throughout the patient-physician relationship. Every physician must decide how to prevent boundary issues from being broken within their own practice. Professional associations such as the American Medical Association may assist in educating, but it must always be the individual physician who sets the standard. By setting high ethics and strong mores, the medical profession ensures that the public will maintain their long-standing trust and an enduring respect for physicians.

Disruptive or Problem Behaviors

Although they do not have a true psychological or health problem, physicians with disruptive or problematic behavior will often find themselves in difficulties with medical or hospital associations or other regulatory agencies. Disruptive behavior can present itself in many forms and may include unacceptable language, bizarre personal habits, abusive or seductive manners, or dissension-producing attitudes. Other examples of physician problematic behavior include repeated unavailability when on call, outbursts or tantrums, insensitivity to women or minorities, and an unwillingness to appropriately communicate or cooperate.

> **Case Vignette.** A physician while making rounds stops at the nursing station. It is the day of his team's big, important football game! The physician, in an attempt to make sure that all present know his loyalties, drops his pants and shows his boxer shorts, done in team colors, complete with team nickname and mascot. He fails to appreciate the looks of surprise and horror on the faces of hospital staff and passing patients and their family members.

Such behavior in the past, although insensitive and crass, may have been acceptable, but the rules have definitely changed. This type of disruptive behavior can be offensive and may very well be reported.

Physicians generally have skills, positions, and authority that have caused them to be held in great esteem by society. They are intelligent, powerful, comparatively autonomous people who are accustomed to directing others. Doctors are not used to being scrutinized and analyzed, especially when it comes to their behavior.

When physicians confront a crisis, they often will appear to be in control. Physicians have developed these skills out of necessity to cope even when under utmost stress. Behavior expectations have changed dramatically in today's more examined professional environment. Behaviors once acceptable, although coarse, no longer are the norms. Many more complaints come to medical associations and state licensing boards from a more demanding public. Doctors with problematic or disruptive behavior may very well be competent and caring, but they are falling into disfavor with colleagues, administrators, state medical boards, and other regulatory agencies and bodies.

There are many causes for problematic behavior. Medicine is and will remain a very high-stress occupation. Stress can come from litigation, domestic conflict, money problems, and changes in the health care system, with their associated increased demoralization, or even from an incessant need by the physician to work both long and hard. Today's medical environment may lead to a physician having low self-esteem, lack of confidence, poor interpersonal skills, and lack of communication capabilities. Behavior problems may be associated with health problems, such as an alcohol or drug dependency, depression, grief, or even a personality disorder. General medical illnesses such as diabetes, thyroid disorders, or other neurologic disorders have also been known to be associated with disruptive behavior.

When physicians are identified with a disruptive or problematic behavior, a constructive approach toward those so afflicted by those in supervisory capacities should be initiated. But for a physician to confront another physician is not easy. Doctors are not trained to do this, and physicians have been taught to respect each other's autonomy. A troubled physician, however, needs to be approached and directed toward an assessment that can deal with the problematic and disruptive behavior in both a positive and a corrective way. Through comprehensive evaluation, specific recommendations can be formulated that can initiate a corrective action plan, preserving the physician's practice in a positive way. An important part of treatment for corrective behavior is to remember that, in general, these are not problematic physicians, but physicians who have developed problematic behaviors.

Physician Criminal Behavior

When physicians commit crimes and are subsequently convicted, this may have a direct impact on their licenses to practice medicine. Although many of the crimes that are committed by physicians occur away from the practice of medicine, society has placed a certain trust in physicians. Society expects physicians to be conscientious and honest in all aspects of their lives. If physicians are convicted of felonies, they may well lose their medical licenses and their privileges to practice medicine, depending upon the findings at the investigations and hearings before state licensing boards. As physicians choose to enter into the practice of medicine, they must realize that they have a received a significant public trust and must continue throughout their career to conduct their lives in a trustworthy manner.

Conclusion

Physicians with medical or psychiatric health problems or with problematic behaviors can be helped only through cooperation and appropriate forms of care. Regulatory agencies, such as state medical boards, medical societies, and associations, hospitals, and other health care providers must work together, not only to benefit the patients but also to assist and help ill physicians. No one benefits when a mentally or physically ill physician remains untreated. Physicians with alcohol or drug dependencies should feel comfortable to come forth and be treated by a caring, nonjudgmental, and helpful medical community. Through concerted efforts, genuine caring and a common trust, physicians with impairments from emotional, psychiatric, and physical health problems as well as drug and alcohol dependencies will be treated and helped. Only then will the healer truly be healed.

Suggested Readings

AMA Board of Trustees Report Y. Physician Ingestion of Alcohol and Patient Care (Resolution 137, I-90);1990.

Blondell RD. Impaired physicians. *Primary Care.* 1993;20:209-219.

Fleming MF. Physician impairment: options for intervention. *Am Fam Phys.* 1994;50:41-44.

Harbison JD. New law avoids unnecessary punishment of impaired physicians. *Minn Med.* 1994;77:41-44.

Ikeda R, Pelton C. Diversion programs for impaired physicians. *West J Med.* 1990;152:617-621.

Irons R. Sexually addicted professionals: contractual provisions for re-entry. *Am J Prev Psychiatry Neurol.* Spring 1991;3:57-59.

Miles S. Do state licensing procedures discriminate against physicians using mental health services? *Minn Med.* 1997;80:42-43.

Morrison J, Wickersham P. Physicians disciplined by a state medical board. *JAMA.* 1998;249:1889-1893.

Myers MF. Treatment of the mentally ill physician. *Can J Psychiatry.* 1997;42(suppl insert).

Pasquale AC, Brian RN. Medical discipline: dealing with physicians who are unscrupulous, disabled, and/or incompetent. *NY State J Med.* 1979;79:1018-1028.

Report of the Ad Hoc Committee on Physician Impairment. Euless, TX: The Federation of State Medical Boards of the United States, Inc. April, 1995.

Report on Sexual Boundary Issues from the Ad Hoc Committee on Physician Impairment. Euless, TX: The Federation of State Medical Boards of the United States, Inc; April 1996.

Texas Medical Association, Committee on Physician Health and Rehabilitation. *Substance Abuse Among Physicians: A Guide for Medical Students, Residents, and Practicing Physicians.* Austin, TX: Texas Medical Association; 1996.

Wise TN. Depression and fatigue in the primary care physician. *Primary Care.* 1991;18:451-464.

Appendix

Open letter from the *Utah Medical Bulletin* by Joseph G. Cramer, MD, President of the Utah Medical Association:

"I am a physician, and president of the Utah Medical Association. I have a wonderful wife and handsome family. I have a good practice, and great partners. I also have depression. I realize as I tell my colleagues in a public way there will be varied responses. Some of you, my fellow physicians, will understand. To others it will be tantamount to a pronouncement of moral inferiority or mental leprosy or marital divorce. And the shunning begins— not because anyone is especially mean; it is just that there are few Miss Manner suggestions on the etiquette of depression. Others will say it is none of their business. To you less serotonin challenged, there is also a great possibility that you won't get it."

"I am informing my friends, my respected peers, and total strangers, linked together as we are all physicians, because I am truly concerned for members of this profession and particularly of this Association. If physicians do not care for other physicians then who will? I personally am fine, and have a very good 'paid friend.' I currently take an SSRI and acknowledge that it may be for the long haul. But I'm thinking of others."

"Medicine is hazardous duty with increasingly less combat pay. The people controlling the dollars are demanding shared risk, but at the same time they have no clue the risks we bear as physicians."

"Medicine can be dangerous business. In the state of Utah in the last 10 years many of our associates have taken their own lives. Of the 200 physicians who have died during the past 10 years in Utah, 5% have been by their own hand."

"A doctor is twice as likely to commit suicide in Utah than the general population. Nationally the suicide rate is 11/100,000. In Utah it bumps up to 14/100,000. For physicians in Utah it approaches 30/100,000!"

"Why are we so deadly? I suppose there is a preselection process of some of us who enter medicine. Maybe some of us are caring or sensitive to a fault. There is the skill and accessibility. If we know how to save lives, we are also capable to end them. There is also the vulnerability of never knowing enough in a profession that demands that we know everything. Expectations and pressures of life and death add to the burden. There is the professional pride that teaches we can not do wrong. Increasing social isolation contributes to the mix. We used to meet in our county and specialty societies, now we are all so busy that the therapy of conversation is declining."

"As I exit the closet of secrecy for mood disorders I ask that each of us examine our own happiness, worries and fears, and have the courage to discover ourselves. We doctors must reflect on the admonition of holy writ, 'Physicians heal thy self.'"

"Let us begin to recognize mood disturbances in ourselves, in our loved ones and our friends. For me silence, anger and irritability were the main features. Others might have other complaints, unrelenting self-criticism, fatigue, lack of interest, familial discord, or troubles at work including substance misuse. Still others may just be afraid. Make the tough decision, seek proper professional or pastoral care. It is okay to be an imperfect human being who happens to practice medicine. Let us do a better job of diagnosing depression in our patients and treating them appropriately or referring properly. Let us work to inform the public that just like diabetes, asthma, and high cholesterol are not signs of weakness in character, the disorders of the central nervous system are based in the science of receptors, neurotransmitters, genetics, family dynamics and personal choices. Let us also make effort to teach the keepers of the purse so that economic parity with other evidence-based specialities becomes a reality."

"Would I have wanted it any different? I do regret any hurt my family may have suffered, but the insights I have gained and the knowledge that I now possess I believe could not have been gained in any other fashion. This editorial is not an offer for us to come down, and all join hands and sing 'Kumbaya', but it is an invitation to the members of this Association to be concerned for others around us, including our fellow doctors and ourselves."

Joseph G. Cramer, MD
President, Utah Medical Association

Chapter 14

Physician Life and Career Health and Development

Todd Pearson, MD

A physician's life and career are necessarily linked, because they cannot be compartmentalized or separated from one another. If life dimensions outside of career are experiencing "disease" or are out of balance, they will affect the health of the physician's career. That the physician's work has a dramatic effect on the health of his or her life dimensions outside of work is a given, especially considering the number of hours spent in the work realm, the nature of the work, the degree to which he or she identifies with his or her work role(s), and the substantial investment he or she has placed in the profession (temporal, financial, emotional, psychological). In turn, the quality of the physician's life and career influences his or her physical, mental, emotional, and spiritual health. The health of the physician's life and career also has a reciprocal relationship with his or her life and career beliefs and practice paradigms. One's biography and beliefs and one's "stories" and paradigms influence one's life and career health just as do genetics and the environment. It is no surprise then that, as the biography and beliefs of physicians are being challenged and rescripted, so too is their life and career health.

The Life/Career Development Needs of Physicians

In my work with individual physicians, medical practices, and health care organizations, a number of patterns of life/career development themes have emerged. These broad themes are as follows:

- individual and organizational renewal
- life/career resilience and strategically linking resilience to academic and corporate business goals
- life/work balance and strategically linking work, life, and family issues to the academic and corporate agenda
- reclaiming soul and spirit (individual and organizational)
- community (developing a deeper sense of meaning, connection, relationship, and belonging).

Within these broad themes, a recurring pattern of specific life/career development needs for physicians have also emerged and are listed in Table 14-1 (page 230).

The Principles of Life/Career Resilience

In the current era of change and complexity, new mental models are required for addressing the life/career health of physicians. The approach to life/career health for physicians should not follow the traditional medical model, which is machine-like (treat the symptoms and fix the broken parts), nor should it be event-driven. Nor should it follow the traditional paradigm that states that the absence of life/career dis-ease or symptoms equates to health. In a health care environment where change is continuous, physicians need to cultivate resilience in order to thrive, be effective, and be fulfilled in their work and career. Resilience is a characteristic that applies equally to physicians who are experiencing relative stability and harmony in their life/career and to those who are suffering from life/career adversity.

Table 14-1
Recurring Life/Career Development Needs for Physicians

- ☐ Examining identity/sense of self
- ☐ Examining sources of security and self-esteem
- ☐ Identifying interests, passions, energizers
- ☐ Exploring personal style, natural rhythm, and preferences
- ☐ Exploring temperament and personality characteristics
- ☐ Identifying dependable strengths, motivated skills, innate talents, and natural gifts
- ☐ Identifying work content, technical, functional, and transferable skills
- ☐ Clarifying values
- ☐ Clarifying the roots of life/work/career stress, dissatisfaction, disaffection, and burnout
- ☐ Assessing life/work/career and physician/work/organizational mismatches
- ☐ Exploring the nature of "calling," one's spirituality, life purpose, and meaning
- ☐ Creating alternative and future-oriented scenarios
- ☐ Addressing work/life/family balance issues
- ☐ Doing values-based currency management—time, money, talent, and energy
- ☐ Examining paradigms, expectations, and attitudes in life, work, career, and practice
- ☐ Learning about chaos, change, transition, and renewal
- ☐ Examining control and autonomy issues
- ☐ Examining will, choice, and commitment
- ☐ Cultivating creativity
- ☐ Cultivating empowerment, optimism, proactivity, hope, trust, and appreciation
- ☐ Reducing disempowerment, pessimism, negativity, hopelessness, fear, externalization, blame, and victimization
- ☐ Identifying realistic and compelling life/work/career options
- ☐ Identifying barriers to change
- ☐ Identifying supports and resources
- ☐ Overcoming isolationism and fostering connections to others
- ☐ Addressing health/self-care needs—physical, mental, social, emotional, and spiritual
- ☐ Cultivating traditional career management strategies
- ☐ Developing a continuous life/work/career learning and unlearning agenda

Life/career resilience is a lifelong personal commitment to manage proactively—from the inside out—one's life, career, and learning in an environment where continuous change is the status quo. This definition includes some of the following tenets:

- it is a lifelong ongoing process
- it is more about enjoying and managing the quality of the life/career journey than it is about "arrival" or a destination to be reached

- it is a state of consciousness and a way of being, employing mindfulness and requiring nonjudgmental intention and attention in present time
- it is a discipline, a practice that must be nurtured and cultivated with the same care, compassion, and commitment as one's medical practice
- it is based on wellness, fitness, and a preventive life/career health model
- it is a "whole-person" approach, taking into account all aspects of one's life, not just work or vocational concerns
- it recognizes the reciprocal interconnection of one's life and work to physical, mental, emotional, and spiritual health
- it embraces the realm of mind, body, and spirit, behavioral medicine, psychoneuroimmunology/endocrinology, and the effects work environments have on life/career health
- it is a "whole systems" approach to life/career, realizing the interconnectedness and interdependence of the multiple systems to which one relates
- it revolves around finding meaning, purpose, commitment, values, integrity, and a sense of identity and community from the inside out

The Characteristics of Life/Career Resilience

Some of the "qualities of being" of a physician who practices life/career resilience are described below.

Self-awareness. Resilient physicians know their core values, interests and passions, preferences, and strengths (VIPS). Self-awareness also includes knowing and embracing one's shadow side, limitations, and weaknesses for the inherent lessons within. In knowing who they are, they have an awareness of where, what, how, and with whom they do their best clinical and nonclinical work. They have clarity regarding the work that is meaningful and satisfying to them and provides the blessing of service to others.

Values Driven. Resilient physicians have clarity regarding their core values and use them to give direction and meaning to their life/career. There is an important and dynamic relationship between physicians' values and those of the practice, groups, and organizations in which they work and spend most of their time. A large inventory of values fall within each of the following four areas, and each value has a meaning unique to the individual:

- intrinsic values – which motivate one to truly love one's work on a daily basis
- work content values – which make one's work activities most satisfying and engaging
- work environment values – which relate to the working conditions that provide an optimum environment to do one's best work
- work relationship values – which are the characteristics of interaction with others in the workplace that are most important to you.

Purpose Driven. The convergence of being self-aware and values driven creates the power of purpose. Purpose provides an internal compass that creates alignment and congruency between who one is and what one does; among mind, body, and spirit; and among thoughts, feelings, and behavior. Purpose provides meaning, an internal sense of control, and a means by which the physician can seek to align with congruent health care delivery systems and practice settings.

Connected. Resilient physicians develop and maintain a personal and professional network of relationships for learning, support, feedback, accountability, and sharing (of ideas, resources, experiences, and feelings). They cultivate meaningful connections in order to accomplish their work, meet goals (personal, professional, and organizational), succeed in their careers, and serve as a buffer to stress and career burnout. Life/career health has more to do with a network of personal and professional belonging and a sense of community than with a position, title, the tools of one's specialty, income, status, or other external sources of perceived security, identity, and self-esteem.

Commitment to Continuous Learning. Commitment to continuous learning is what separates the proactive from the reactive or inactive. It is a way to keep pace with the speed of change. Most physicians are committed to keeping up to date clinically and are now increasingly asked to acquire skills in the nonclinical realm. Some of these skills are shown in Table 14-2.

Table 14-2
Nonclinical Skills Being Asked of Physicians

- ☐ Life skills
- ☐ Technology skills
- ☐ Work strategy/relationship skills
- ☐ Career management skills
- ☐ Values-based time and financial management skills
- ☐ Corporate management/managed care skills
- ☐ "Unlearning skills"

Examination of Paradigms. Paradigms are mental models, assumptions, scripts, perceptions, attitudes, and expectations; they are ways of viewing our life/career and the outside world. Resilient physicians have an awareness of how their paradigms and their ways of thinking and feeling shape their experiences. Many physicians are trapped by old paradigms and old "rules," while resilient physicians are able to create synergy between the "old" and the "new."

Vision. Resilient physicians practice the art of the long view, designing compelling, realistic, future-oriented scenarios for growing their life, work, and career. They are adept at scanning the horizon for trends and benchmarking best life/career practices that are in alignment with who they are and who they are becoming.

Change Hardy. Change is a global reality that shapes and defines our lives, leveling the playing field, and creating new needs, interfaces, and opportunities. Resilient physicians anticipate, understand, and adapt to change, using change as a resource and consciously viewing transitions as part of a life/career path of personal and professional learning and discovery.

Balance. Resilient physicians live a life of equilibrium unique to them in a way that reflects their values and what provides meaning and fulfillment. This includes balancing their "being" and "doing"; their multiple roles, commitments, activities, and obligations; their mind, body, emotions, and spirit; their critical currencies of time, money, talent, and energy; and the past, present, and future. At core, they realize that balance is essentially about the wholeness in which all the dualities, polarities, and complementary forces in their lives/careers find resolution.

Practice. Resilient physicians maintain a consistent "practice" of taking time for reflection and contemplation, a daily commitment to develop intention and consciousness. It is a grounding tool and centering strategy for self-knowledge, discovery, tapping one's intuition, and accessing one's heart. Common "practice" activities include silence and solitude, contemplative prayer, keeping a journal, spending time alone in nature, walking, running, other forms of solo exercise, meditation, breathing practices, yoga, tai chi, aikido, chi-gong, etc.

Appreciation. Resilient physicians practice gratitude and appreciation even in down times, harboring a positive outlook and operating from a position of abundance, faith, and trust as opposed to scarcity and fear. They appreciate and reflect on what delights them, what surprises them, what is going well, or what they have to be grateful for. They have the capacity to notice and acknowledge the presence of things for which they yearn and are able to discern these things in incomplete states or in packages and places they do not expect. They appreciate the power within the daily and the ordinary.

Physician Career Adversity Syndromes

The current drivers and emerging trends in health care have all conspired to create major paradigm shifts for the physician's world of work. A massive change in the numbers, types, and skills required of health care professionals is under way. We are experiencing dramatic alteration in who delivers care to whom and where, when, and how that care is delivered. We are seeing changes in specialty mix, roles, responsibilities, status, and compensation. The sequelae of these drivers and trends produce potentially disabling stress, manifested by an increase in physical problems and illness, increasing difficulty with relationships, increased negative thoughts and feelings, an increase in maladaptive coping behaviors and habits, and exhaustion.

With increasing frequency we are witnessing physician career adversity syndromes (PCASs), listed in Table 14-3. These include the states of burnout, rustout, and disaffection. These three entities often predispose to or abet the other PCASs I commonly refer to as "the D's": disability, dependence, disruptive/dysfunctional behavior, disciplinary action, disengagement, and displacement. There is overlap in the PCASs, and one may predispose to another. They are intertwined, and many physicians suffer from more than one of these syndromes, either simultaneously, sequentially, or on a recurring basis. Several indicators suggest an increased prevalence in PCASs (Table 14-4). Some of the more common factors causing career burnout, rustout, and disaffection and predisposing to the other PCASs are listed in Table 14-5.

Table 14-3
Physician Career Adversity Syndromes

☐ Burnout
☐ Rustout
☐ Disaffection
☐ Disability
☐ Dependency/impaired
☐ Disruptive/dysfunctional behavior
☐ Disciplinary action
☐ Disengagement
☐ Displacement

Table 14-4
Indicators that Suggest Increasing Incidence of PCASs

- ☐ Trends in the physician disability insurance industry
- ☐ Trends in malpractice insurance industry
- ☐ Predictions by futurists and career development specialists
- ☐ Work/career satisfaction surveys and published reports
- ☐ Career burnout surveys and published reports
- ☐ Life/work balance surveys and published reports
- ☐ Out-migration to nonclinical or nonmedical careers and early retirement
- ☐ The incidence of disruptive/dysfunctional physicians and assessment programs for same
- ☐ License revocations, suspensions, surrenders, and disciplinary actions/reprimands
- ☐ The changing nature of impaired physician profiles and physician health programs
- ☐ The physician as employee
- ☐ Involuntary unemployment/underemployment for new resident graduates
- ☐ Involuntary unemployment/underemployment for practicing physicians
- ☐ Physician oversupply and workforce projections
- ☐ The use of nonphysician clinicians and extenders in health care
- ☐ The use of alternative/complementary medicine providers
- ☐ Unionization and collective bargaining

Table 14-5
Factors Causing or Predisposing to PCASs

- ☐ The combination of emotionally taxing work, a strong service orientation, and being patient centered
- ☐ Reaching a normal disenchanted phase of work/career development
- ☐ Life components out of balance
- ☐ Failing to set appropriate limits
- ☐ Old or incomplete beliefs and practice paradigms
- ☐ Working in an unpleasant or "toxic" environment
- ☐ Being a "vulnerable host" (ie, less "immune" secondary to genetics or predisposing personality characteristics)
- ☐ Lacking work that matches core values, interests/passions, preferences/personality, dependable strengths/motivated skills
- ☐ Work overload, both qualitative and quantitative
- ☐ Lack of participation, control/autonomy, choice, and options (perceived and real)
- ☐ Insufficient rewards, recognition, and appreciation (perceived and real, intrinsic and extrinsic)
- ☐ Lack of respect, openness, trust, and fairness in relationships
- ☐ Breakdown in community, loss of collegiality

Description of the PCASs

Burnout. Career burnout, as it is traditionally defined, is a syndrome resulting from prolonged chronic stress. It is usually paired with high expectations and emotionally taxing work. It is a cumulative process that occurs over time and results in physical, emotional, and mental depletion. It is characterized by the development of a negative self-concept and negative attitudes toward life, work, career, and other people. The somatic manifestations of this condition have been well documented. The emotional manifestations fall within two dimensions. The first dimension is characterized by *cynicism* and includes feelings of negativity, victimization, resentment, entrapment, and behaviors of externalization that are reactive and often disruptive or dysfunctional. The second dimension is characterized by *withdrawal* and includes feelings of isolation, hopelessness, helplessness, disempowerment, disillusionment, being "stuck," and behaviors of disengagement. The mental manifestations include maladaptive behaviors and coping techniques such as substance abuse and/or other addictions and compulsivity syndromes.

Work addiction is the socially acceptable form of addiction within our culture that claims both primary and secondary victims. Other mental manifestations of workplace stress and burnout include depression and other primary affective or nervous/anxiety-related disorders. Chronic overstress leads to the three classic stages of burnout:

- *Exhaustion* – affected individuals are overextended emotionally, physically, and mentally. They have nothing left to give, are drained, are used up, and lack energy. Paradoxically, they often are unable to unwind, relax, or recover.

- *Depersonalization* – affected individuals are often cold and distant toward work and people. They minimize their involvement to protect themselves from further compromise and depletion. They don't have the time or interest to be with others and tend to withdraw and isolate themselves. They may manifest the behaviors that come with cynicism.

- *Ineffectiveness and a decreased sense of personal accomplishment* – in this last stage, affected individuals tend to trivialize or harbor feelings of "hollow victories" and "empty laurels." They suffer from a loss of passion, purpose, and creativity. They lack confidence in their ability to make a difference and harbor a sense of inadequacy (the "imposter syndrome"). They feel everything is overwhelming, become increasingly ineffective, and have difficulty with decision making.

Case Vignette. Dr R is a 54-year-old pediatrician who would like to pursue early retirement. She admits she would probably not be entertaining retirement if it were not for the current health care environment. She is having to work harder for less in the way of both psychic and financial rewards. She is feeling the stress of decreased autonomy and increased accountability, liability, and responsibility as a primary care practitioner. She does not find as much joy in patient care as she once did, and she laments the loss of collegiality and sense of community she once felt with her peers. She finds that she increasingly has difficulty enduring the rigors of call. She recently was named in a malpractice suit, her first, regarding a patient for whom she was only peripherally involved. Her name has become part of the public record and she is undergoing all the elements inherent in malpractice stress. During the last few years she has experienced migraine headaches with increasing frequency and recently was placed on antihypertensive medication for elevated blood pressure. She knows these are work stress-related health problems. She states that she has no concept of her identity beyond being a pediatrician and explains that her family, finds much of their identity and sense of security with her being a physician as well. She is the primary breadwinner for her family and her two children are approaching college age. She is concerned for her health and feels trapped, scared, and without options.

Rustout. This is a variation of burnout. It is the deterioration or degeneration of ability and character that results from inactivity, neglect, or misuse. It is caused by staying in one place or doing the same thing for too long, or it is due to a lack of variety, challenge, and intellectual stimulation. It can occur if there is not ample opportunity to use one's preferred talents and motivated skills, pursue one's preferred passions and interests, work with and within one's preferred communities of interest, or a combination of these. If extreme or chronic, it can lead to all the manifestations of burnout. Unlike burnout, which tends to wear on the individual from the presence of chronic overwhelming external conditions, rustout is more of an "inside-out" process. It is caused by the lack of creative tension or "positive" stress; the presence of tasks whose completion hold little intrinsic meaning and are not linked to one's sense of purpose; and/or the lack of tasks that do add intrinsic meaning to one's life.

Disaffection. Career disaffection refers to the gradual erosion of contentment that comes with a loss of loyalty and allegiance to a given work, career, organizational, or professional setting. It involves a sense of alienation, especially when the workplace, organization, or leadership does not behaviorally model the values it supposedly espouses. It occurs if there exists a mismatch between the individual's core values, expectations, and standards of practice and that of the organization(s) and systems with whom they interface. Career disaffection is integrally related to burnout, and one can lead to the other.

If these three syndromes are allowed to progress unchecked, the affected physician may progress to develop one of the problematic "D" conditions.

Disability. The frequency of disability claims filed by physicians during the 1990s has skyrocketed. There are several reasons for this, but there is no denying a correlation to the changing work environment and its impact on physicians. The nature, severity, and duration of disability claims have also experienced change. Career disaffection, burnout, and rustout can predispose to acute ailments or exacerbate chronic medical conditions that lead to disability. This relates to multiple factors—environmental, biologic, psychologic, emotional, spiritual and social—that conspire to adversely affect health. The nature of disability claims now includes an increased prevalence of conditions known to be associated with stress, such as depression, emotional-behavioral disturbances, nervous and anxiety-related disorders, gastrointestinal disorders, cardiovascular disorders, back ailments, arthritis, autoimmune disorders, and chronic fatigue.

Career dissatisfaction, disaffection, and burnout also contribute to decreased commitment to continue with one's medical work or to find creative ways to work around an existing medical condition. In some instances there may exist a disincentive to work when a physician can earn the same income or more on disability than in working in his or her field. And if the physician is dissatisfied in his or her work and career and he/she perceives alternative career options to be limited, the duration of disability claims may also be prolonged.

Case Vignette. Dr P has been practicing emergency medicine for 15 years. During the last two years he has endured burnout, depression, and chronic low back pain. During a recent 12-hour shift he exacerbated his low back problem and subsequently was found to have a ruptured lumbar disk. He is considering filing for disability but is concerned about how his peers and family may react. He is frightened and confused as to his options. All he knows is what he dislikes and no longer wants in his work/career. Beyond that he does not have a clue as to who he is, what he could do, or what resources are available to help him. He feels both confined and defined by the initials "MD" that are behind his name.

Dependence/Impairment. The nature of impairment is also changing and now includes more stress-related disorders that impair work performance and competence. These may or may not be associated with the comorbidity of abuse or dependency. Dependence and impairment are often linked with the other PCASs, especially disability, disruptive behavior, and disciplinary action.

Case Vignette. Dr L is an anesthesiologist who recently was "diverted" to a physician health program for chemical dependency. He also suffers from a coexisting bipolar disorder. As part of his intervention, reentry, and aftercare program he was referred for life/career coaching to better ascertain what environment and options would be most congruent with who he is and what is important to him in his life/career. He embarked upon a process of self-assessment. He explored his personal and professional identity, his core values, and the values that held the most meaning for him in his work. He examined his temperament, personal style, and preferences within the work environment. He became more familiar with his dependable strengths, motivated skills, and innate talents— many of which were not being utilized in his day-to-day clinical duties. He discovered that his passions and interests, within both medicine and life, were not being tapped. He also discovered how out of balance his life had become and came to realize who he was as a "whole person" and how this had been compromised prior to his entry into the diversion program.

Disruptive/Dysfunctional. This refers to a constellation of aberrant interpersonal behaviors and misconduct that adversely affect the health care workplace and patient care. There is an increased incidence of reports for physicians with disruptive and dysfunctional behavior. In part, this is because of less tolerance for, and an increased awareness of, this syndrome. It is also a direct reflection of the stressors within the health care workplace and their impact on the individual physician. The disruptive physician often manifests coexistent PCASs.

> **Case Vignette.** Dr M is a prominent cardiologist well known within both the academic and clinical ranks. He has been under increasing stress in his practice and is feeling burned out. He is working longer and harder and has seen his income drop 20% during the last two years. He considers the health care organization for which he works to be a "toxic" work environment. During the last year he has increasingly been verbally abusive with staff, colleagues, and patients. After losing his temper and throwing a scalpel during a procedure in which the proper equipment was not available, he was placed on probation and given an ultimatum to attend a multidisciplinary professional assessment program for physicians. Although "vocational rehabilitation" was offered as a part of his assessment program, he also sought coaching on his own for a more holistic assessment of his life/career, and to address his growing questions and concerns about work/career "fit" and to what degree his career disaffection and disruptive behavior were a reflection of the dysfunctional environment in which he worked and was expected to return. This became both an individual and an organizational consultative process. The organizational component focused on improving the workplace environment and its systems and processes, and on providing enduring longitudinal resources for the employee's life/career health.

Disciplined. A small but significant proportion of physicians are disciplined each year for a variety of offenses. The more frequent serious offenses include negligence or incompetence, substance abuse, inappropriate prescribing practices, inappropriate contact with patients, and fraud. The increasing incidence of license revocations, suspensions, and surrenders may well result from increased awareness, education, and reporting, combined with less tolerance for these behaviors.

Disengaged. This refers to physicians who have "resigned without resigning" and do the absolute minimum to survive and get by within their environment. Their primary purpose to practice is a paycheck, and their sense of meaning and fulfillment is found outside the work realm. They are the "dead wood" within practices and organizations. This syndrome also includes those who exhibit a variation of "short-timer's syndrome," those who are disengaging from clinical medicine because of their unhappiness and who may or may not have a sense of future career direction. This may include many from the ranks of those considering early retirement or those moving to alternative work arrangements such as part-time status, job sharing, and sabbaticals. This PCAS often includes productive and talented individuals whose frustration and pain threshold exceeds their internal or external incentives to continue in clinical medicine.

Displaced. This refers to those individuals who have been involuntarily displaced for a variety of reasons that are often out of their control. They may be unemployed or underemployed in their field of specialty. Displacement can result from downsizing; loss of patient base or dismissal for not meeting performance, productivity, quality, utilization, or other standards; restrictive covenants or no-compete clauses; practicing in a low-demand and/or overpopulated specialty and/or exclusionary medical environment (ie, areas of high managed care penetration and hypercompetition); job loss because of merger, acquisition, failed health care organization, or venture; being an international medical school graduate who has completed residency training in the United States; being inappropriately stigmatized for a PCAS that does not affect competence (discrimination); or other forms of discrimination (lifelong or long-standing disabilities, gender, sexual orientation, ethnicity/race, age, etc).

Significance of the PCAS

Career burnout merits special attention because of its epidemic increase within our profession; the myths and misconceptions surrounding its cause and therefore its prevention, intervention, and treatment; and because it is the one PCAS that is most likely to precipitate and/or be associated with the others. Each person expresses career burnout in a unique way, but the basic themes are the same. It most typically occurs in physicians who are by all external standards considered to be rising toward or at the height of their career. These are individuals experiencing the erosion of human soul, the starvation of spirit, the loss of will, a conflict in core values, and a sense of compromised integrity—integrity to self, significant relationships, patients, and what provides meaning in their work. They are struggling with their personal and professional identity and sense of purpose, the stressors of the workplace, and the new paradigms relative to work/career in medicine. This conceptualization of burnout transcends the prevailing focus on personality and the emotional-psychological self, a focus that fails to adequately address the existential and spiritual dimensions.

The PCASs reflect a "gap" that comes at a human price. They reflect the distance between the physician and the demands of the job and workplace. They reflect a chronic imbalance in which the physician's work/career demands more than the physician can give and provides less than the physician needs. They measure the disparity between expectations and reality and the void between who we are and what we do. They represent the gap between economic values and human values and reflect work settings in which human values come in second to economic ones. This includes human values such as what inspires and provides meaning to the physician's work life. The PCASs are an important barometer of social, organizational, professional, and cultural dysfunction in the workplace.

Conventional wisdom and focus have primarily been on the PCAS being a problem of the individual. The physician is said to suffer from flaws in character, constitution, hardiness, behavior, and personality. These flaws are purported to be genetically predisposed or in some way reflect a lack of ambition and "fitness." In fact, this is less a matter of "survival of the fittest" (the John Wayne School of Medicine) than it is "survival of that which fits best." But because the PCASs are visible at the individual level—in terms of health, emotions, and behavior—a traditional medical model has been employed that focuses on the individual physician. This model stigmatizes, pathologizes, and stresses characterologic shortcomings, and finds its solution in fixing, changing, or dismissing the individual. The focus has been on improving coping skills, perception management, attitude, and learning to live with the way things are. Considerable evidence, however, emphatically argues that the primary problem lies within the environment in which they work. Increasingly the PCASs say more about the conditions of the job, existing structures and systems, and the functionality of the health care workplace than they do about the individual physician. If the workplace does not reflect the human side of our work, the human side of change, there is a significant risk of career burnout and other PCASs and the high price they carry.

The current model is equivalent to treating symptoms without diagnosing and treating root causes, or focusing on a part without seeing the dis-ease of the whole. In my experience, it is frequently the most committed, idealistic, dedicated, and creative physicians, the "star performers" and "high potentials," who are most likely to burn out while being thwarted by the dysfunctional systems and environment in which they work. Indeed, the most "stress-hardy" physician will succumb to burnout in a "toxic" work environment that predisposes to same.

Warning Symptoms and Signs

These descriptions and vignettes illustrate some of the symptoms and signs that should urge physicians to take heed, wake up, and pay attention to their life/career health. There exist both internal and external cues that suggest one is at risk for the PCASs (see Table 14-6). Internal cues are those that fall within the physical, mental, emotional, and spiritual domains, while external cues are signals that come from the feedback and reactions received from the environment. In interpreting these cues, it is important to ascertain whether there are recurring patterns that require attention and to step outside of one's self, ego, defenses, and personality to find symbolic meaning and learning that could facilitate constructive change for the better in one's life/career.

Table 14-6
Individual Clues Indicating Risk for PCASs

Internal cues

☐ Physical – somatic manifestations associated with chronic or excessive stress

☐ Emotional – nature of predominant feelings and behaviors expressed in life/work/career

☐ Mental – problematic predominant thoughts, maladaptive coping behaviors and techniques, decreased sense of personal accomplishment

☐ Spiritual – existential concerns

External cues

☐ Workplace – feedback and reactions from peers, superiors, staff, patients, and others

☐ Important relationships – feedback and reactions from spouse, significant others, family, friends, coworkers

☐ Health care marketplace – feedback from local, regional, and national drivers, trends and events that affect work/career circumstances, goals, and needs

As with individuals, there are also warning symptoms and signs within organizations that herald the workplace as one that adversely affects life/career health. These are cues to the presence of organizational factors that may contribute to the development of PCASs (see Table 14-7).

Table 14-7
Organizational Clues Indicating Risk for PCASs

☐ Poor satisfaction surveys

☐ Perceived negative public image of the practice or institution

☐ Flat or decreased productivity

☐ Individuals remain outliers when measured against peers in spite of consistent, timely, and appropriate feedback in performance reviews

☐ Decreased morale, commitment, engagement, and work satisfaction (observed, surveys)

☐ Dysfunctional communication patterns, relationships, and teamwork

☐ Preexisting high incidence of PCASs

☐ Frequent downsizing/rightsizing

☐ Frequent budget cuts

☐ Difficulties in recruitment and retention

☐ High incidence of stress-related illness, worker's compensation, and absenteeism

☐ High incidence of out-migration to early retirement and nonclinical/nonmedical careers

☐ High incidence of requests for alternative work arrangements – part-time, job share, flex time, sabbaticals

☐ Frequent meetings and policy changes to deal with the fallout from all of the above

Prevention

Individual Responses

Life/career health requires self-efficacy and is the individual physician's responsibility. Toward this end, some suggestions to facilitate the prevention and early intervention of the PCASs include the following:

- Adapt the core principles, characteristics, qualities of being, and mindset for life/career resilience outlined above
- Develop a continuous personal and professional development plan that will address
  - the characteristics of life/career resilience that require growth
  - personal life/career development needs (Table 14-1)
  - personal factors that may predispose to the PCASs (Table 14-6)
  - the fit among self, the nature of the work, and the workplace
  - the presence of both internal and external cues of career disease

In implementing a development plan, one should prioritize action steps based on degree of importance, commitment (the likelihood of actual follow-through), and control (which steps and hoped-for outcomes are within the individual's sphere of influence). Before implementing these steps, it may be helpful to borrow from the Pareto principle utilized in quality improvement, ie, isolate and focus upon root causes to life/career disease (80% of the problem is caused by 20% of the causes).

Some of resources physicians can seek to facilitate their life/career resilience are included in Chapter 15. Other resources include the following:

- seeking "intentional" role models and mentors who possess qualities the physician desires to incorporate into his or her life/career
- connecting with other physicians and tapping into the power of community

- attending seminars, workshops, retreats, in-services, conferences, and keynote presentations on topics related to one's life/career development needs and life/career health

- accessing the many books, audiotapes and videotapes, and multimedia and Internet resources pertinent to the development of life/career resilience and the prevention or intervention of the PCASs.

- utilizing the other tools, techniques, strategies, and practices suggested elsewhere within this book

Although life/career resilience can be developed in a self-directed manner, there is much to recommend the guidance of a qualified life/career development professional.

System Responses: Academic, Corporate, and Organized Medicine Approaches

The traditional definitions and approaches to career burnout and the other PCASs are not wrong, but they are incomplete. Frequently their cause lies more within the work environment and are a reflection of dysfunction or fundamental change within the workplace and in the nature of the physician's work. Below are some suggestions for our practices, organizations, organized medicine, and the multiple other stakeholders in health care who have a vested interest in life/career resilience for physicians.

- employing the principles, characteristics, and "qualities of being" espoused in life/career resilience for individuals. Each characteristic has an organizational equivalent. "Resilient" organizations that practice these principles will be more successful in attracting and cultivating "resilient" individuals

- adopting a preventive life/career health model for physicians, seeing them as vulnerable human beings working within environments that have factors that predispose toward these syndromes

- acknowledging the importance of the essence and integrity of the human spirit

- addressing the links between "toxic" work environments and life/career disease and applying it to the health care workplace

- identifying and remedying mismatches among the physician, the nature of his or her work, and the workplace environment and its culture. The provision of orientation and mentoring programs and annual reviews separate from performance reviews can help facilitate this

- developing strategies drawn from virtuality, learning organizations, systems thinking, evidence-based best practices, and continuous quality improvement. Some ways to achieve this include the Internet and intranets; tapping the intellectual capital and creativity within the organization to pursue personal, professional, and organizational goals; and isolating root causes and implementing core solutions to dysfunctional organizational environments, systems, structures, processes, and cultures that may predispose to the PCASs.

- creating "people development" plans that acknowledge and address the life/career development needs of their physicians

- organized medicine and health care organizations should seek strategic alliances both within and outside of the health care industry to help support and fund research and education for physician life/career health issues

- incorporating life/career resilience for physicians across the medical training lifespan continuum, taking an approach to prevention and intervention as an ongoing, longitudinal "process"

It is both an opportunity and a responsibility for our health care organizations and organized medicine to invest in the creation of a life/career resilient physician workforce. This implies providing ongoing education, resources, systems, processes, time, tools, vehicles, and strategies for physicians to "own" their life/career resilience and for the early intervention and prevention of PCASs. Indeed, there exists a strong business case for incorporating life/career resilience processes to achieve corporate business goals and for linking these initiatives to the academic/corporate health care agenda (Table 14-8). It provides a "win-win" process that aligns the needs of both physicians and the health care organizations through which they interact and/or are employed. In the future, resilience will be the most important sustainable competitive advantage in the marketplace for physicians, for health care organizations, and for the provision of quality patient care that they both desire.

Table 14-8
The Business Case for Investing in the Prevention of PCASs

☐ Decreased costs associated with:
 – recruitment, retention, turnover, staff shortages, training and orientation
 – out-migration to nonclinical/nonmedical careers and early retirement
 – low morale, commitment, loyalty
 – poor teamwork, collaboration, communication, and relationships
 – problematic practice style, referral patterns, efficiency, effectiveness, productivity, adherence to guidelines, and performance standards
 – absenteeism
 – stress-related illness, worker's compensation
 – risk management/claims reduction – workplace harassment, discrimination, disruptive/dysfunctional behavior, liability/malpractice, impairment, disciplinary action
 – clinically adverse events and errors that do not result in litigation
 – intervention/treatment programs and severance packages
☐ Beneficial effects on mentoring programs, leadership development, succession planning, and "star" performers/high potentials
☐ Improved patient satisfaction, public image/perception, perceived quality of care
☐ Increased satisfaction of managed care organizations, employers with whom patient care contracted, insurers, etc

Summary

There are powerful economic, political, social, and technologic forces affecting the nature of our work, our medical workplaces, our organizations, and the profession as a whole. These forces are affecting all stakeholders in health care. The solution to the human fallout we are experiencing from this needs to look at the health care workplace, organizational environments and their cultures, the medical profession and its culture, and the individual. PCASs impact the individual, relationships, organizations' practices, the health care workplace, the profession, and society. There are multiple reasons, economic and otherwise, for all stakeholders in health care to invest in life/career resilience and the prevention and amelioration of the PCASs.

Chapter 15

Resources

Roger Brown, PhD,
Larry S. Goldman, MD

I n general, the first resource to which physicians or others should turn is the state physician health program. Nearly every state medical society sponsors or is associated with a program that is designed to assist physicians who are in need of assistance or about whom there are concerns. Some state programs have programs to provide assistance to physicians or their families to ensure that treatment is available. State programs vary in terms of the types of assistance they offer: all address issues of addiction, many handle other psychiatric or behavioral problems, and some deal with physical illness, stress, family problems, and so on. State society programs also vary in terms of their reporting and other relationships with the state licensing boards; many programs are strong advocates in licensing board actions for physicians receiving care in their programs. All programs can be contacted anonymously and information obtained (eg, referrals) without disclosing identifying information. All of the state medical society programs are listed later in this chapter.

Another source, frequently overlooked, is the state medical licensing board or authority. In addition, a number of medical specialty societies have committees dealing with health-related issues that may be of assistance to their members. These may be at the national or state level.

Also included in this chapter are a variety of other resources that might be either useful or of interest. These include:

- Various private groups that deal with particular issues
- A listing of sources for additional general information on substance abuse and physically disabling conditions
- Groups sponsored by professional societies for dentists, pharmacists, veterinarians, and attorneys

Not included in this chapter are private chemical dependency and other treatment programs for physicians. These programs are not included for two reasons. First, many states have relationships with particular treatment programs, and a physician in need of treatment would be well advised to consult with his/her state program in order to facilitate recovery and ensure continued licensure. Second, on a more practical level, these programs are subject to change, with facilities opening, closing, and reaffiliating regularly.

Please note that the inclusion of these resources does not imply any endorsement by the American Medical Association (AMA). These groups are included solely for the information of interested readers.

The **Federation of State Physician Health Programs** (FSPHP), which is the national umbrella organization for the individual state society programs, regularly produces a directory of all of these programs with detailed, state-by-state listings of many specific program elements. Information about the FSPHP and its directory can be obtained from AMA's physician health program at 515 North State Street, Chicago, IL 60610; phone 312 464-5066; fax 312 464-5841.

State Physician Health Programs

Alabama Physicians Recovery Network
19 South Jackson Street
Montgomery, AL 36104
334 261-2044, 334 261-2006 fax
800 239-6272

Physicians Assistance Committee
Alaska State Medical Association
PO Box 230630
4107 Laurel Street
Anchorage, AK 99508
907 276-2474, 907 276-2462 fax

Arizona State Medical Society
Physicians Health Program
1651 East Morten Avenue, Suite 210
Phoenix, AZ 85020-4624
602 331-1073 or 255-4161
602 255-1848 fax

Physicians Health Committee
Arkansas Medical Foundation
23157 I-30, Suite 201
Bryant, AR 72022
501 847-8088, 501 847-7130 fax

California Physician Diversion Program
1420 Howe Avenue, Suite 14
Sacramento, CA 95825
916 263-2600, 916 263-2607 fax

California Medical Association
Committee on the Well-Being of
Physicians
221 Main Street, PO Box 7690
San Francisco, CA 94120-7690
415 882-5189

Colorado Physician Health Program
899 Logan Street, Suite 505
Denver, CO 80203
303 860-0122, 303 860-7426 fax

Connecticut State Medical Society
Physician Health Program
160 St. Ronan Street
New Haven, CT 06511
Norbeckmt@aol.com
203 865-0587, 203 865-4997 fax

Physicians' Health Committee
Medical Society of **Delaware**
1925 Lovering Avenue
Wilmington, DE 19806
302 658-7596, 302 658-9669 fax
info-msd@medsocdel.org

Physician Health Program
2215 M Street, NW
Washington, **DC** 20037-2059
202 466-1800, 202 466-1845 fax

Physicians Recovery Network
Impaired Practitioners Program of
Florida
PO Box 1881
Fernandina Beach, FL 32035-1881
904 277-8004, 904 261-3996 fax
800 888-8776

Physicians Well-Being Program
Medical Association of **Georgia**
PO Box 279
Hinesville, GA 31310
912 884-2686, 912 884-5018 fax

Hawaii Medical Association
Committee on Physicians Health
1360 South Beretania Street, 2nd Floor
Honolulu, HI 96814
808 536-7702

Idaho Physician Recovery Network
Physician Health Program
PO Box 2668
Boise, ID 83701
208 344-7888, 208 344-7903 fax

Illinois State Medical Society
205 West Touhy
Park Ridge, IL 60068
847 698-4722, 847 698-4907 fax
Triathdoc@aol.com

Indiana State Medical Association
Physician Assistance Program
322 Canal Walk
Indianapolis, IN 46202-3252
317 261-2060, 317 261-2076 fax
cbacker@ismanet.org

Physician Recovery Program
Iowa Board of Medical Examiners
1209 East Court Avenue
Des Moines, IA 50010
515 281-5171, 515 242-5908 fax

Medical Advocacy Program
Kansas Medical Society
623 SW 10th Avenue
Topeka, KS 66612-1627
800 332-0156, 913 235-5114 fax

Kentucky Physicians Health
Foundation – Impaired Physicians
Program
9000 Wessex Place, Suite 305
Louisville, KY 40222-8512
502 425-7761, 502 425-6871 fax

Louisiana Physician Health Program
Louisiana State Medical Society
6767 Perkins Road
Baton Rouge, LA 70808
504 763-8500 or 800 375-9508
504 763-6122 fax

Physician Health Program
Maine Medical Association
PO Box 190
Association Drive
Manchester, ME 04351
207 623-9266, 207 622-3332 fax

Medical and Chirurgical Faculty State
of **Maryland**
Physician Rehabilitation Program
1204 Maryland Avenue, 2nd floor
Baltimore, MD 21201-5512
800 992-7010, 410 962-5583 fax

Physician Health Services, Inc
A **Massachusetts** Medical Society
corporation
1430 Main Street
Waltham, MA 02154
617 893-4610 or 800 322-2303
617 893-5321 fax

Michigan State Professions
Recovery Program
PO Box 989
Brighton, MI 48116
810 225-1350, 810 225-1358 fax

Minnesota Medical Association
Minnesota Physician Support Services
3433 Broadway Street, NE., #300
Minneapolis, MN 55413-1761
612 362-3761, 612 378-3875 fax

Caduceus Club of **Mississippi** Inc
2600 River Ridge Road, Suite 203
Jackson, MS 39216-5013
601 981-3408, 601 981-3475 fax

Missouri Physicians' Health Program
3839 Lindell Boulevard
St. Louis, MO 63108
314 371-5225, 314 652-6033 fax
msma.mphp@sprintmail.com

Missouri Alternate
MAOPS – Physician Health Program
1125 Madison
Jefferson City, MO 65102
573 636-8255, 573 636-7505 fax

Montana Professional Assistance
Program
1242 North 28th Street, Suite 222
Billings, MT 59101
406 245-4300, 406 245-4432 fax

Nebraska Medical Association
Impaired Physicians Program
233 South 13th Street, Suite 1512
Lincoln, NE 68508-2091
402 474-4472, 402 474-2198 fax

Southern **Nevada** Physicians' Assistance
2590 East Russell Road
Las Vegas, NV 89120
702 739-9034, 702 739-6345 fax

Nevada Alternate
State Diversion
Nevada Health Professionals Foundation
665 Skyline Boulevard
Reno, NV 89509
702 742-1171 or 258-8969
702 258-8967 fax

Physician Health Program
New Hampshire Medical Society
7 North State Street
Concord, NH 03301
603 226-3494, 603 226-2432 fax

Impaired Physicians Program
Medical Society of **New Jersey**
2 Princess Road
Lawrenceville, NJ 08648
609 896-1766, 609 896-1884 fax

New Mexico Monitored Treatment
Program
9204 Menaul NE, Suite 6
Albuquerque, NM 87112
505 271-0800, 505 271-1914 fax

Committee for Physicians' Health
Medical Society of the State of
New York
99 Washington Avenue, Suite 1111
Albany, NY 12210
518 436-4723, 518 436-7943 fax

North Carolina Physicians Health
Program
4700 Six Forks Road, Suite 220
Raleigh, NC 27609
919 881-0585, 919 881-0505 fax

North Dakota Physicians' Health
Program
North Dakota Medical Association
PO Box 1198
Bismark, ND 58502-1198
701 223-9475, 701 223-9476 fax

Ohio Physicians Effectiveness
Program, Inc
445 East Granville Road
Building C
Worthington, OH 43085
614 841-9690, 614 891-1050 fax

OSMA Physician Recovery Program
Oklahoma State Medical Association
601 West I-44 Service Road
Oklahoma City, OK 73118
405 376-9786 or 843-9571
405 376-1831 fax

Oregon Diversion Program for
Health Professionals
6950 SW Hampton Street, Suite 220
Tigard, OR 97223-8331
503 620-9117, 503 684-5512 fax

Physicians Health Programs
Pennsylvania Medical Society
777 East Park Drive
PO Box 8820
Harrisburg, PA 17105-8820
717 558-7750, 717 558-7818 fax
php-trust@mamedsoc.org

Associación Médica de **Puerto Rico**
Impaired Physicians Committee
PO Box 9387
San Juan, PR 00908-9387
809 721-6969, 809 722-1191 fax

Physicians' Health Committee
Rhode Island Medical Society
106 Francis Street
Providence, RI 02903
401 331-3207, 401 751-8050 fax

Physicians Advocacy and Assistance
Committee
South Carolina Medical Association
PO Box 11188
Columbia, SC 29211
803 798-6207, 803 772-6783 fax

South Dakota State Medical
Association
Impaired Physicians Program
1323 South Minnesota Avenue
Sioux Falls, SD 57105-0685
605 336-1965, 605336-0270 fax

Physicians Health Program
Tennessee Medical Foundation
PO Box 1317
Murfreesboro, TN 37133-1317
615 893-7755, 615 890-2096 fax

Committee on Physician Health and
Rehabilitation
Texas Medical Association
401 West 15th Street
Austin, TX 78701-1680
512 370-1342, 512 370-1636 fax
linda_k@texmed.org

Physicians Health Committee
540 East 500 South
Salt Lake City, **UT** 84102-2784
801 355-7477, 801 532-1550 fax
utahmed@xmission.com

Vermont State Medical Society
Impaired Physicians Program
136 Main Street, Box H
Montpelier, VT 05601
802 223-7898, 802 223-1201 fax

Physicians' Health and Effectiveness
Program
4205 Dover Road
Richmond, **VA** 23221
804 353-2721, 804 355-6189 fax

Virgin Islands Medical Society
Impaired Physicians Program
PO Box 1490 Christiansteve
St. Croix, VI 00821
809 778-5305, 809 778-5100 fax

Washington Physicians Health Program
720 Olive Way, Suite 525
Seattle, WA 98101
206 583-0127, 206 583-0418 fax

West Virginia State Medical Association
Impaired Physicians Program
4307 Mac Corkle Avenue, SE
Charleston, WV 25364
304 925-0342, 304 925-0345 fax

Statewide Physician Health Program
State Medical Society of **Wisconsin**
PO Box 1109
Madison, WI 53701
608 257-6781, 608 283-5401 fax
soniap@smswi.org

Wyoming Professional Assistance
Program, Inc
231 South Wilson
Casper, WY 82601
307 265-3791, 307 265-4480 fax

Career Counseling Resources

The **Center for Physician Renewal** is devoted to the facilitation of life/career resilience for health care professionals and the creation of "resilient" health care organizations. The Center is a coaching and consultative resource for individuals, groups, and health care organizations and strives to meet the needs of those with growing questions and concerns regarding life/career fit. Center personnel work with physicians experiencing stress, burnout, disenchantment, or displacement in their work/career. A significant portion of work is with individuals and health care organizations wishing to be proactive and avoid these conditions. The Center does this through individual coaching/consultation, group facilitation (seminars, workshops, presentations, retreats, etc), public speaking, writing, and organizational coaching/consultation. The Center for Physician Renewal is located in Bellevue, Washington. Contact Todd Pearson, MD, 10900 NE Fourth Street, Suite 2300, Bellevue, WA 98004; phone 253 351-8577; e-mail mdrenew@aol.com.

The following career counseling resources have been compiled by Dr Pearson:

Colorado Personalized Education
for Physicians
10800 East Bethany Drive, Suite 275
Aurora, CO 80014
Attn: Elizabeth Korinek, MPH,
Director
Voice 303 750-7150;
Fax 303 750-7171

Oregon Medical Association
Individualized Physician Renewal
Program
5210 Corbett Avenue
Portland, OR 97219
Attn: Laurel Case, MD, Director
Voice 503 226-1555;
Fax 503 241-7148

State University of New York
Department of Family Medicine
Health Science Center at Syracuse
475 Irving Avenue, Suite 200
Syracuse, NY 13210
Attn: William Grant, EdD, Director
Voice 315 464-6997;
Fax 315 464-6982

East Carolina School of Medicine
Clinical Enhancement Program
4n-78 Brody Medical Sciences
Building
Greenville, NC 27835-4353
Attn: Stephen Willis, MD, Director
Voice 919 816-2601;
Fax 919 816-3040

University of Wisconsin Medical
School
Department of Continuing Medical
Education
2715 Marshal Court
Madison, WI 53707
Attn: Thomas Meyer, MD
Voice 608 263-2852;
Fax 608 262-8421

The **Center for Professional and Personal Renewal** offers support and revitalization to health care professionals. Workshops for individuals and couples, individual coaching, and consultation to organizations are available. Contact Dr Peter Moskowitz at 555 Bryant Street, Suite 160, Palo Alto, CA, 94303, 800 377-1096 or 650 329-0297, pmoskowitz@batnet.com.

MD CareerNet provides career planning and management resources for physicians, focusing on assisting physicians who are interested in broadening their career paths beyond patient care. Assistance is given to help physicians establish themselves as part-time consultants or full-time employees in nonpatient care roles in industrial settings (eg, pharmaceuticals, biotechnology, information technology, and medical devices). Physicians can seek a confidential career consultation for a range of types of concerns, including a desire to stay in clinical medicine but enhance the quality and balance of one's life; establish greater financial earning power; renew their passion about their work; establish a creative outlet within their professional life; develop and market a niche area of expertise as a consultant; leave patient care and transition into another sector of the health care market; plan a sabbatical or retirement; or develop a new product or business. Contact Gigi Hirsch, MD, 183 State Street, 6th Floor, Boston, MA 02109; phone: 617 227-2115; fax 617 227-6954; www.mdcareer.net; e-mail ghirsch@mdcareer.net.

The **AMA** publishes a book, *Leaving the Bedside: The Search for a Nonclinical Career*, for physicians considering or needing to leave clinical practice. The book, revised in 1997, reviews different options, aids in personal self-assessment, and helps development of an action plan. It may be ordered from AMA publications, asking for order #OP392096AIJ. Current prices are $25.95 for AMA members and $32.95 for nonmembers. The AMA has also published a document entitled, *Closing Your Practice: 7 Steps to a Successful Transition*, which explains many of the steps involved in doing so. Either book may also be ordered by phone, 800 621-8335, or via the AMA Web site, www.ama-assn.org.

The **Medical Forum** is a career guidance program based in the United Kingdom and run by Dr Sonia Hutton-Taylor. Their Web site (www.fast.to/medicalforum) has information for physicians thinking about career changes.

Wellness Organizations

The **Center for Professional Well-being** is a nonprofit educational organization devoted to promoting well-being and preventing stress among professionals, student professionals, and family members. These goals are accomplished through various educational, consulting, and advisory programs and services. The Center publishes a quarterly Bulletin, *Being Well*; sponsors intensive retreats; provides scholarships for needy professionals; and promotes networking among individuals and groups who support quality-of-life interventions. Small groups and individuals can receive intensive educational intervention and well-being advice. Off-site services include the conduct of retreats for groups or practices, educational lectures and seminars, and consulting services. Contact John-Henry Pfifferling, PhD, Director at the Center for Professional Well-being, 21 West Colony Place, Suite 150, Durham, NC 27705; phone 919 489-9167; fax 919 419-0011; www.cpwb.home.mindspring.com; e-mail CPWB@mindspring.com.

Other Physician-Related Resources

The **American Medical Association Alliance** has a number of publications that may be of interest to concerned spouses and other family members. Of particular interest is the pamphlet, *What Every Physician's Spouse Should Know*, which deals with stress and substance abuse. Write the Alliance at 515 North State Street, Chicago, IL 60610.

The Elsa Barton Scholarship provides educational assistance to spouses or dependents of impaired physicians. It is supported by the **American Psychiatric Association Auxiliary**. Call Charlotte Wilson at 619 259-5582 for information.

There are well-established physician health committees or resources at the **American Psychiatric Association,** the **American Society of Anesthesiology,** the **American College of Physicians/American Society of Internal Medicine,** the **American College of Surgeons,** the **American Academy of Physical Medicine and Rehabilitation,** and the **American Society of Addiction Medicine.** In addition, the **Association for Academic Physiatry,** an organization of teachers of rehabilitation medicine, has developed guidelines for medical schools to use in assessing applicants and students with physical disabilities.

Physicians Against Latex Sensitization (PALS) is a not-for-profit organization for physicians who are committed to halting the growing epidemic of latex allergy. It is headed by Barbara Zucker-Pinchoff, MD, an anesthesiologist in practice for 13 years, now disabled by latex allergy. The group is dedicated to sharing knowledge about latex allergies. They can be reached at bzpmd@aol.com or at the PALS Web site (www.pals.net).

A general resource for those physicians or trainees with physical disabilities is **The American Society of Handicapped Physicians,** 3424 South Culpepper Court, Springfield, MO 65804, 417 881-1570 (contact Ms Jericho Peden).

International Doctors in Alcoholics Anonymous (IDAA) has compiled a list of its members who will serve as resources for state or local medical societies, specialty societies, or medical schools interested in alcoholism among physicians. Contact Dr Richard McKinley at IDAA, PO Box 199, Augusta, MO 63332, 314 482-4548 for information.

The **Center for Professional Health** at Vanderbilt is a new training resource to assist physicians with problems resulting from misprescribing of drugs. Contact Dr Spickard at 615 936-0678 for more information. Other similar programs can be found at Case Western Reserve University, University of Kentucky, and Mercer University (Georgia).

Aid for Impaired Medical Students (AIMS) is a program in several medical schools designed to help students struggling with addictions. Contact Dr Patrick Wahl, who runs the program at the University of Tennessee in Memphis, 901 448-5686, for information about the program and other sites.

General Health Resources of Interest to Physicians

Substance Abuse and Psychiatric Disorders

Alcoholics Anonymous
www.alcoholics-anonymous.org

National Institute on Alcohol Abuse and Alcoholism (NIAAA)
www.niaaa.nih.gov

National Institute on Drug Abuse (NIDA)
www.nida.nih.gov

National Institute of Mental Health (NIMH)
www.nimh.nih.gov

Substance Abuse and Mental Health Services Administration (SAMHSA)
www.samsha.gov

Physical Disabilities and Injuries

The **Alexander Graham Bell Association for the Deaf** is a nonprofit membership organization that was established in 1890 to empower persons who are hearing impaired to function independently by promoting universal rights and optimal opportunities to learn to use, maintain, and improve all aspects of their verbal communications, including their abilities to speak, speech read, use residual hearing, and process both spoken and written language. Alexander Graham Bell Association for the Deaf, 3417 Volta Place, NW, Washington, DC 20007-2778, www.agbell.org

National Institute on Disability and Rehabilitation Research (NIDRR) is a unit within the Office of Special Education and Rehabilitative Services (OSERS) of the US Department of Education and provides leadership and support for a comprehensive program of research related to the rehabilitation of individuals with disabilities. www.ed.gov/offices/OSERS.

National Institute of Neurological Disorders and Stroke, www.ninds.nih.gov

National Stroke Association, www.stroke.org

In order to assist the 7,800 individuals who sustain a spinal cord injury each year, and the 400,000 persons living with spinal cord injuries, the **National Spinal Cord Injury Association** was established in 1948. The Association serves not only persons with spinal cord injuries but also persons who have diseases or conditions, the effects of which are similar to those of spinal cord injuries, for examples, multiple sclerosis. www.spinalcord.org

Other Related Professional Organizations

The **American Dental Association** (ADA) Well-being and Assistance Programs offer confidential assistance for dentists and/or their concerned family members. Dentistry can be stressful and poses unique challenges and risks to its practitioners. When personal problems arise, dentists often do not want to seek help and try to cope on their own. The Well-being and Assistance Program helps dentists at the first sign of problems, with the goal of assisting the dentist toward optimum health while maintaining the ability to continue professional practice or to return to practice. ADA Council on Dental Practice, Dentist Well-being and Assistance Program, 211 East Chicago Avenue, Chicago, IL 60611, www.ada.org/prac/wellbe.html

American Pharmaceutical Association's (APhA) Pharmacy Recovery Program, established in 1982, fosters the development and strengthening of state- and campus-level programs to assist pharmacists and pharmacy students whose competence has been compromised by the disease of chemical dependency or by other causes. APhA Pharmacy Recovery Network, 2215 Constitution Avenue, Washington, DC 20037, www.aphanet.org

To provide a model for assisting lawyers whose practices had been impaired by addictions, the **American Bar Association** created the Commission on Impaired Attorneys in 1988. In August 1996, its name was changed to the Commission on Lawyer Assistance Programs (CoLAP) in order to describe better the Commission's expanded services to include stress, depression, and other mental health problems and to avoid any stigma that its former name may have implied. Its primary goal is to advance the legal community's knowledge of impairments facing lawyers and its response to those issues. All 50 states have developed lawyer assistance programs or committees focused on quality-of-life issues. These programs employ the use of intervention, peer counseling, and referral to 12-step programs to assist in the lawyer's recovery process. American Bar Association, Commission on Lawyer Assistance Programs, 750 North Lake Shore Drive, Chicago, IL 60611, www.abanet.org/cpr/colap/home.html

American Veterinary Medical Association has a Wellness Committee and a Chemical Impairment Program for veterinarians. www.avma.org

Index

D

Defense mechanism, 41

Denial, 41, 88

Dependency, 240-241

Depression, 80-81

administrative responses to, 214-215

anxiety and, 81-82

biological risk factors, 83

defenses, 87-88

diagnosis, 87

in medical, law and graduate students, 43

open letter about, 225-227

preventing, 92-93

psychological risk factors, 84-85

social risk factors, 86

trainees and, 165

treating, 88-92

Dickstein, Leah J., 1-7, 161-176

Dietary habits, physicians', 12

Dilts, Stephen J., 118-135

Disabilities. *See* Physical disabilities, physicians with

Disability claims, 239-240

Disaffection, 239

Disengaged physicians, 242

Displacement, 88, 242-243

Disruptive behaviors, 241

administrative responses, 221-223

managing physicians with, 145-147

personality disorders and, 141-145

Dissociative identity disorder, trainees and, 169

Diversion programs, 3, 211

Drug use, intimate relationships and, 57-58

Dual doctor couples, 69-71

Due process, 209

Dysfunctional behaviors, 241

Dysfunctional family legacies, 171-172

E

Eating disorders, trainees and, 168

Elsa Barton Scholarship, 258

Exercise habits, physicians', 12

F

Federation of State Physician Health Programs (FSPHP), 251

Female physicians. *See* Women physicians

4 D's of mis-prescribing, 216

Frank, Erica, 9-16

G

Gautam, Mamta, 80-93

Gay male physicians/trainees

relationships and, 72-74

stress issues for, 174-175

Gendel, Michael H., 118-135, 138-158

Goldman, Larry S., 1-7, 193-203, 250-262

Goldstein, Marion Zucker, 180-191

Grief, unresolved, 170-171

H

Hand functions disabilities, diminished, 23

Handicapped physicians. *See* Physical disabilities, physicians with

Harassment. *See* Sexual harassment

Hartman, David, 26-27

Health screening practices, physicians', 12

Hearing impairment, 24

HIV/AIDS, 212

Humor, black, 41

S

Sexual contact, with patients, 148-149
  legal and ethical aspects of, 149-151
Sexual harassment, 156
  of women trainees, 173
Sexual improprieties, 218
Sexual misconduct. *See* Sexual violation
Sexual transgression, defined, 149
Sexual violation, 217-221
  case examples of, 153-158
  classifications of, 151-152
  defined, 149
Sick doctor statutes, 1
"Sick Physician, The" report (1972), 1-2
Silverman, Morton M., 95-113
"Slippery slope" concept, 150, 153-154
Smoking, cigarette, 11
Special needs, physicians with. *See*
Physical disabilities, physicians with
State physician licensing boards, 207-209
Stetten, DeWitt, 35
Strax, Thomas E., 17-37, 26
Stress
  lawsuits and, 66-67
  managing, and recovering physicians,
  130
  on physicians, 41-44
  for trainees, 169-173
  women physicians and, 44-50
Students, medical. *See* Trainees
Sublimation, 88
Substance abuse
  early studies of physicians and, 2
  resources for, 260
Substance Abuse and Mental Health
Services Administration, 260

Substance use disorders (SUDs), 157
  course of, 118-121
  diagnosis, 123-124
  evaluation, 122-124
  identification of, 121
  intervention, 121
  regulatory issues and, 130-135
  treating, 124-128
  work-related issues and, 128-130
Suicide, 95-96
  consequences of, 109-110
  female physician, 104
  future research on, 110-111
  incidence of, 96-101
  medical trainees and, 105
  preventing, 108-109, 113
  psychiatric disorders and, 106-107
  rates, 102-104
  risk factors, 107-108, 112
  role strain and, 105-106
  specialties and, 104-105
  in specialty areas, 104-105
  trainees and, 165-166
Suicide studies
  case definition in, 99
  methodological problems with, 97-99
  statistical issues with, 99-102